T0334276

Cases in Haematology

A solid grounding in and understanding of haematology is crucial for any doctor. The pathophysiology is fascinating, and the pharmacology is rapidly advancing, improving prognosis across many haematological conditions. Getting to grips with its fundamentals will stand any medical student in good stead during undergraduate studies and on into clinical practice.

This book utilises single best answer-style questions in the popular *MasterPass* series of revision aids, covering the haematology presentations and conditions listed in the Medical Licensing Assessment content map, making it ideal for MLA preparation and a useful case-based learning resource for any medical student working towards qualifying examinations.

MasterPass Series

Neurosurgery: The Essential Guide to the Oral and Clinical Neurosurgical Exam, 2E
Vivian Elwell, Ramez Kirollos, Syed Al-Haddad, Peter Bodkin

Sport and Exercise Medicine: An Essential Guide
David Eastwood, Dane Vishnubala

Clinical Consultation Skills in Medicine: A Primer for MRCP PACES
Ernest Suresh

Refraction and Retinoscopy: How to Pass the Refraction Certificate, 2E
Jonathan Park, Leo Feinberg, David Jones

The Final FRCA Constructed Response Questions: A Practical Study Guide, 2E
Elizabeth Combeer, Mitul Patel

Diagnostic EMQs: A Comprehensive Collection for Medical Examinations
Syed Hussain, Umber Rind, Jawed Noori, Yasmean Kalam, Haseeb Ata and Emanuel Papageorgiou

Passing the Final FFICM: High-Yield Facts for the MCQ & OSCE Exams
Muzzammil Ali

Cases in Haematology: For the MLA and PLAB
Aaron Niblock

Postgraduate Ophthalmology Exam Success
Maneck Nicholson, Anjali Nicholson, Syed Faraaz Hussain

Pass the MRCP (SCE) Neurology Revision Guide
Dhananjay Gupta

For more information about this series please visit:
https://www.routledge.com/MasterPass/book-series/CRCMASPASS

Cases in Haematology

For the MLA and PLAB

Aaron Niblock
Haematology Consultant
& Senior Clinical Lecturer
School of Medicine
Ulster University
Northern Ireland

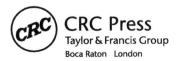

CRC Press
Taylor & Francis Group
Boca Raton   London

CRC Press is an imprint of the
Taylor & Francis Group, an **informa** business

Designed cover image: Shutterstock image – 251299024

First edition published 2025
by CRC Press
2385 NW Executive Center Drive, Suite 320, Boca Raton FL 33431

and by CRC Press
4 Park Square, Milton Park, Abingdon, Oxon, OX14 4RN

CRC Press is an imprint of Taylor & Francis Group, LLC

ISBN: 9781032817590 (hbk)
ISBN: 9781032817576 (pbk)
ISBN: 9781003501190 (ebk)

DOI: 10.1201/9781003501190

Typeset in Helvetica Neue
by Apex CoVantage, LLC

'Education is not the filling of a pail, but the lighting of a fire.'

William Butler Yeats, 1865–1939

CONTENTS

CONTENTS

PREFACE

Understanding haematology is crucial for any doctor. The pathophysiology is fascinating, and the pharmacology is rapidly advancing, improving prognosis across many haematological conditions. Getting to grips with its fundamentals will stand you in good stead during your clinical years. This book utilises single best answer questions, making its structure and layout perfect for the United Kingdom Medical Licensing Assessment (MLA). The book covers the haematology presentations and conditions listed in the MLA content map.

The clinical-based questions are followed by answers explaining the key physiological principles, allowing the reader the knowledge to answer similar styled questions.

The concluding section is a test yourself section with single best answers testing the knowledge you have gained.

We hope this book prepares you for the upcoming exam and wish you every success in your career.

ACKNOWLEDGEMENTS

Professor Denis Alexander (DPhil, FRCPath) has had a long career in NHS haematology, where he practised at the interfaces between diagnosis, research and clinical practice. He also has had a decades-long association with Ulster University as Visiting and Part-Time Lecturer, Visiting Professor, Professor and, since 2015, with Stratified/Personalised Medicine. He has over 100 publications cited in PubMed. Until recently, he was an examiner at the Royal College of Pathologists (London) and has served as an external examiner for primary and higher degrees in several universities, including as Opponent for Public Defence of several PhD theses at Uppsala University in Sweden. He has been instrumental in his encouragement of medical staff in research for which I am forever thankful.

The illustrations throughout the book have been done by my daughter, Evie, whose natural talent is evident.

ABOUT THE AUTHOR

Dr Aaron Niblock graduated from Queens University Belfast in 2008; subsequently, he achieved Membership to the Royal College of Physicians (MRCP London) and was later awarded FRCP.

He gained his FRCPath in haematology, thereafter completing an MSC with distinction in cancer and molecular pathology and genomics at Barts and The London. He has also completed the European Haematology Exam.

Currently, Dr Niblock is working as a consultant haematologist and senior clinical lecturer in the Ulster University School of Medicine.

In his medical career, he has published in numerous peer-reviewed journals and presented nationally and internationally. He continues his academia along with his clinical practice.

ABBREVIATIONS

ACS	Acute coronary syndrome
ADAMTS13	A disintegrin and metalloprotease domain with thrombospondin type 1 motif, member 13
AF	Atrial fibrillation
aHUS	Atypical haemolytic uraemic syndrome
ALL	Acute lymphoblastic leukaemia
ALP	Alkaline phosphatase
ALT	Alanine transaminase
AML	Acute myeloid leukaemia
APL	Acute promyelocytic leukaemia
APTT	Activated partial thromboplastin time
AST	Aspartate transaminase
ATR	Acute transfusion reaction
ATRA	All-trans-retinoic acid
BA	Breathing air
BP	Blood pressure
BPM	Beats per minute
COPD	Chronic obstructive pulmonary disease
CLL	Chronic lymphocytic leukaemia
CML	Chronic myeloid leukaemia
CMV	Cytomegalovirus
cOCP	Combined oral contraceptive pill
Crea	Creatinine
CXR	Chest X-ray
DAT	Direct antiglobulin test
DHTR	Delayed haemolytic transfusion reaction
DIC	Disseminated intravascular coagulation
DOAC	Direct oral anticoagulant
DPG	Diphosphoglycerate
DVT	Deep vein thrombosis
EBV	Epstein–Barr virus
EDTA	Ethylenediaminetetraacetic acid
EMA	Eosin-5-maleimide
EPO	Erythropoietin

ET	Essential thrombocytosis
FBP	Full blood picture
FFP	Fresh frozen plasma
FIB	Fibrinogen
fL	Femtolitre
FNHTR	Febrile non-haemolytic transfusion reaction
g/L	Grams per litre
G6PD	Glucose-6-phosphate dehydrogenase
GFR	Glomerular filtration rate
GGT	Gamma-glutamyl transferase
GH	Genetic haemochromatosis
GSH	Glutathione
GSSG	Glutathione disulphide
Hb	Haemoglobin concentration
Hct	Haematocrit
HE	Hereditary elliptocytosis
H&E	Haematoxylin and eosin
HELLP	Haemolysis, elevated liver enzymes and low platelets
HHV8	Human gamma herpes virus 8
HIV	Human immunodeficiency virus
HL	Hodgkin lymphoma
H. pylori	Helicobacter pylori
HR	Heart rate
HRS	Hodgkin Reed–Sternberg
HRT	Hormone replacement therapy
HTC	Hospital transfusion committee
HTLV	Human T-lymphotophic virus
HTT	Hospital transfusion team
HUS	Haemolytic uraemic syndrome
INR	International normalised ratio
ISI	International sensitivity index
ITP	Immune thrombocytopenia purpura
IV	Intravenous
JVP	Jugular venous pressure
LDH	Lactate dehydrogenase
LMWH	Low-molecular-weight heparin
LRTI	Lower respiratory tract infection
MAHA	Microangiopathic haemolytic anaemia

MALT	Mucosa-associated lymphoid tissue
MCH	Mean cell haemoglobin
MCHC	Mean cell haemoglobin concentration
MCV	Mean cell volume
MDS	Myelodysplasia
MGUS	Monoclonal gammopathy of undetermined significance
MHRA	Medicines and Healthcare Products Regulatory Agency
MM	Plasma cell myeloma
MTX	Methotrexate
NADPH	Nicotinamide adenine dinucleotide phosphate
NHL	Non-Hodgkin lymphoma
NSTEMI	Non-ST-elevation myocardial infarction
O&S	Organisms and sensitivity
PCC	Prothrombin complex concentrate
PE	Pulmonary embolism
Pg	Picogram
PK	Pyruvate kinase
PLT	Platelet
PMF	Primary myelofibrosis
PML RARA	Promyelocytic leukaemia/retinoic acid receptor alpha
PNH	Paroxysmal nocturnal haemoglobinuria
PPI	Proton pump inhibitor
PPP	Pentose phosphate pathway
PT	Prothrombin time
PV	Polycythaemia vera
RCC	Red cell count
RCOG	Royal College of Obstetricians and Gynaecologists
ROTI	Related organ or tissue impairment
RR	Respiratory rate
Sats	Saturation
SCD	Sickle cell disease
SFLC	Serum free light chains
SHOT	Serious Hazards of Transfusion
SVC	Superior vena cava

SVCO	Superior vena cava obstruction
TACO	Transfusion-associated circulatory overload
T°C	Temperature degrees Celsius
TEG	Thromboelastography
TFT	Thyroid function test
TRALI	Transfusion related acute lung injury
TTP	Thrombocytopenia purpura
U&E	Urea and electrolytes
ULN	Upper limit of normal
US	Ultrasound
VTE	Venous thromboembolism
WCC	White cell count
WHO	World Health Organization

MLA CONDITIONS

Adverse drug effects
Anaemia
Arterial thrombosis
Disseminated intravascular coagulation
Epistaxis
Haemochromatosis
Haemoglobinopathies
Haemophilia
Hyposplenism/splenectomy
Leukaemia
Lymphoma
Multiple myeloma
Myeloproliferative disorders
Patient on anti-platelet therapy
Polycythaemia
Pulmonary embolism
Sickle cell disease
Transfusion reactions
Vitamin B12 and/or folate deficiency
VTE in pregnancy and puerperium

part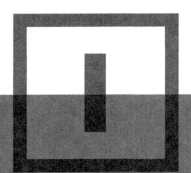

Clinical Cases

section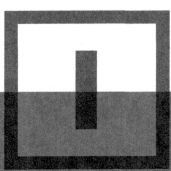

Benign Haematology

Case 1

A 16-year-old woman attends with decreasing energy and poor concentration for a year. She gives a 2-year history of menorrhagia.

On examination, a general pallor is noted, with brittle, spoon-shaped nails.

Bloods:

Hb 52g/L   (120–160)
MCV 66fL   (80–96)
MCH 24pg   (27–33)
WCC 8.1 × 10^9/L   (4.0–11.0)

How is this anaemia classified?

a) Microcytic hypochromic anaemia
b) Microcytic hyperchromic anaemia
c) Normocytic anaemia
d) Macrocytic hypochromic anaemia
e) Macrocytic hyperchromic anaemia

ANSWER CASE 1

Answer: a

The haemoglobin molecule is required to carry oxygen around the body. Some red cells carry more haemoglobin than others; therefore, the concentration of haemoglobin is directly correlated with the oxygen combining capacity. The World Health Organization (WHO) defines anaemia as a haemoglobin concentration or number of red cells lower than normal.

As anaemia results in less oxygenation of tissues, symptoms can include fatigue, weakness, shortness of breath, dizziness and palpitations, amongst others.

Blood cells are made in the bone marrow. This blood-producing factory, if working correctly with adequate delivery of iron, B12 and folate, should produce red cells, white cells and platelets.

The earliest red cell is an erythroblast. This cell is nucleated and grows in islands attached to a macrophage. The erythroblast nucleus develops at the same time as iron is being fed from the macrophage

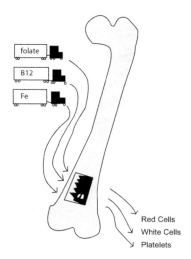

FIGURE 1.1 Image demonstrating the delivery of iron, B12 and folate to the bone marrow factory to allow for the production of red cells, white cells and platelets.

to the globin chains, making haemoglobin in the cytoplasm. Vitamin B12 and folate are required to make thymine nucleotides required for DNA (see Figure 1.1). A shortage of these vitamins results in a delay in nuclear maturation. This delay inadvertently results in more haemoglobin in the cytoplasm, leading to larger cells (macrocytes) but fewer in number. The reverse occurs when the DNA is maturing at a steady rate but there is not enough iron (iron deficiency) or not enough globin (thalassaemia); this results in small red cells (microcytes).

It makes sense that we classify anaemias by the size of the red cells (mean cell volume, MCV), as this gives a clue to the underlying aetiology.

Classification of anaemia

Microcytic	Normocytic	Macrocytic
Iron deficiency	Marrow failure	B12 deficiency
Thalassaemia	Renal failure	Folate deficiency
Sideroblastic anaemia	Anaemia of chronic disease	Hypothyroidism
Lead poisoning		Myelodysplasia
Anaemia of chronic disease		Drugs
		Alcohol

In this case, the anaemia is microcytic hypochromic, and the most common cause worldwide is iron deficiency. The probable cause in this example is menorrhagia. The body recycles iron normally from aged red cells that get removed by the spleen around 120 days. The iron is recirculated back to the macrophage in the bone marrow for new red cells. Unfortunately, if blood loss occurs, this iron is not available and can eventually lead to a net deficiency. The first-line treatment is with oral iron until normalisation of Hb, MCV and MCH, followed by an additional 3–6 months to replete iron stores. There is evidence to support alternate-day iron in the treatment of iron-deficient women. IV iron is licensed in the setting of iron deficiency anaemia with intolerance to oral iron.

Case 2

A 6-month-old presents to the Emergency Department (ED) with hepatosplenomegaly, failure to thrive and a progressive pallor.

Bloods:

Hb 66g/L	(113–141)
MCV 62fl	(70–85)
RCC 4 × 10¹²/L	(4–5.5)
WCC 8.1 × 10⁹/L	(6.0–15.0)

Normal iron stores.

What is the likely cause of this anaemia?

a) Iron deficiency
b) Alpha thalassaemia trait
c) Beta thalassaemia
d) HbH disease
e) Hb Barts hydrops fetalis

DOI: 10.1201/9781003501190-04

ANSWER CASE 2

Answer: c

This case evaluates the understanding of globin chain production.

Through the embryonic, fetal and new-born stages, the haemoglobin molecule changes. It is required to do this, as the affinity of oxygen needs to change as development occurs. In the developing fetus, fetal haemoglobin (HbF, $\alpha 2 \gamma 2$) is dominant, and it has a higher affinity for oxygen than adult haemoglobin (HbA, $\alpha 2 \beta 2$), allowing the fetus to remove oxygen easily from maternal circulation. When the child is born, the dominant haemoglobin type must change to adult haemoglobin, as the priority is to deliver oxygen to all the organs and tissues.

The alpha-chain gene is coded for on chromosome 16 and the beta chain on chromosome 11. Within these genes, there is genetic switching to allow different haemoglobin molecules to be produced.

The alpha chain is fully developed in the fetus and so present at birth. Therefore, if there is a severe abnormality with the alpha chain, for example, HbH, the child is symptomatic at birth. On the other hand, the gamma (γ) in HbF switches to beta (β) in HbA week on week until 6 months of life. Therefore, if a child presents around 6 months, as in this case, the suspicion is that of a β-chain abnormality like beta thalassaemia. HbH and Hb Barts hydrops fetalis both involve the alpha chain and therefore are present at birth. Hydrops fetalis is not compatible with life.

Alpha thalassaemia traits are asymptomatic and therefore would not explain the anaemia.

Case 3

A 28-year-old man with a known history of Crohn's disease presents with shortness of breath going up stairs.

On examination, his complexion is mildly icteric and pale. The sclera is yellow.

Investigations are as follows:

Hb 73g/L   (130–175)
MCV 110fL   (80–96)
Reticulocytes 12%   (1–2%)
WCC 9.2 × 10⁹/L   (4–11)
Platelets 499 × 10⁹/L   (150–400)
Bilirubin 45μmol/L   (<17)

What is the probable cause of this anaemia?

a) Iron deficiency
b) Anaemia of chronic disease
c) B12 deficiency
d) Hypothyroidism
e) Sideroblastic anaemia

DOI: 10.1201/9781003501190-05

ANSWER CASE 3

Answer: c

This macrocytic anaemia is the result of vitamin B12 deficiency. Only 60% of patients with B12 deficiency will have macrocytosis. Vitamin B12-deficient red cells produced are large and fragile. In severe deficiency, some red cells haemolyse as a result; therefore, the haemolytic screen will be positive.

B12 laboratory assays are moving towards active B12 rather than total B12.

The most common cause of B12 deficiency is pernicious anaemia. Intrinsic factor antibodies are very specific, but sensitivity is low. Therefore, the absence of intrinsic factor antibodies does not exclude pernicious anaemia.

As Crohn's disease can inflame the terminal ileum, the site of absorption of B12, this can result in a deficient state.

If B12 and folate are both low, always replace B12 first. As they both share a metabolic pathway, failure to replace B12 will result in a further drop as folate is replaced. Further depletion of B12 can cause subacute degeneration of the cord.

Case 4

A 75-year-old man with a history of urinary retention awaits an appointment with urology. He has noticed over the past 6 months decreasing energy; however, he can still walk 3 miles a day. He has been treated with 3 courses of antibiotics over the past few months for community-acquired pneumonias.

On examination, the cardiovascular system is unremarkable. On abdominal examination, there is no palpable mass or organomegaly.

Bloods:

Hb 76g/L   (130–175)
WCC 2.1 × 10⁹/L   (4–11)
Neutrophils 0.9 × 10⁹/L   (2–7.5)
Platelets 75 × 10⁹/L   (150–400)
CRP <5mg/L   (<5)
Coagulation screen: Within normal range
Blood film: Leucoerythroblastic blood film

What is the likely underlying aetiology?

a) Chronic myeloid leukaemia
b) Disseminated intravascular coagulation
c) Metastatic prostate cancer
d) B12 or folate deficiency
e) Myelofibrosis

DOI: 10.1201/9781003501190-06

ANSWER CASE 4

Answer: c

As the haemoglobin, white cells and platelets are low, this is a case of pancytopenia. The blood film examination has reported a leucoerythroblastic appearance. Therefore, the immature cells that normally exist in the bone marrow have now entered the blood stream. This is a sign that the bone marrow is struggling. The differential diagnosis includes sepsis, but this is unlikely, as the C-reactive protein (CRP) is normal and the patient is stable, awaiting an outpatient review. Therefore, suspicion is that the bone marrow is infiltrated with a pathological process and not allowing enough room for haematopoietic cells. As this man has prostatic symptoms, the suspicion is prostatic cancer that has metastasised to the bones.

Both myelofibrosis and chronic myeloid leukaemia are associated with splenomegaly and the latter more with myeloid proliferation; therefore neutrophilia would be expected. Myelofibrosis has a leucoerythroblastic blood film, although you would also expect to see tear drops.

Case 5

A 16-year-old attends the ED with shortness of breath.

On examination:

Oxygen saturation (Sats) on breathing air (BA) 82%
Respiratory rate (RR) 25
Blood Pressure (BP) 120/80mmHg
Heart Rate (HR) 98 beats per minute (BPM)
Temperature (T°C) 39
CXR: New pulmonary infiltrates

Bloods:

Hb 98g/L   (130–175)
WCC 12 × 10⁹/L   (4–11)
Absolute neutrophil count (ANC) 8 × 10⁹/L   (2–7.5)
Platelets 158 × 10⁹/L   (150–400)
CRP 68mg/L   (<5)

The haematology lab makes contact, informing you that sickle cells and Howell–Jolly bodies are seen on the blood film.

What is the most appropriate initial intervention?

a) Oxygen
b) Blood transfusion
c) Antibiotics
d) Pain relief
e) Hydroxycarbamide

DOI: 10.1201/9781003501190-07

ANSWER CASE 5

Answer: a

Sickle cell disease (SCD) is an abnormality involving the beta chain (ch11). It is a single-point mutation at position 6 when glutamic acid is replaced with valine. When both chromosomes contain the abnormal gene, SCD is present. The substitution results in the globin structure being sensitive to certain triggers. The critical outcome is the reduced solubility of HbS when deoxygenated, compared to HbA, leading to tactoid formation within the red cells and the formation of a rigid, sickle-shaped cells rather than the normal, deformable, biconcave disc shape when the red cell contains HbA. These sickled cells are unable to pass through the microvasculature in, for example, the spleen, leading to painful infarcts and eventual atrophy of the organ. A sickle cell crisis can be triggered by hypoxia, increased CO_2, acidaemia, alcohol, cold temperature, dehydration and infection, resulting in the red cells acquiring an irreversible sickle shape (C-shaped). These events can result in blood vessels being occluded.

Several types of crises can occur:

Splenic sequestration is when blood becomes entrapped in the spleen, resulting in enlargement and pain. This crisis occurs only in children, as the spleen usually undergoes atrophy from recurrent crisis to an asplenic stage by the teenage years.

Acute chest crisis is the leading cause of hospitalisation and death in people. The signs are that of a severe chest infection including fever and chest X-ray (CXR) infiltrates and can be the result of a vaso-occlusive crisis.

Vaso-occlusive crisis is the most common presentation, characterised by severe pain and the result of a complex interaction of the sickle cells and endothelial lining.

Aplastic crisis is when red cell production is inadequate and, in patients with haemoglobinopathies such as sickle cell disorders, the red cell life span is short. Therefore, when erythropoiesis is halted, this can result in a profound anaemia. With sudden drops in haemoglobin without the expected reticulocyte response, acute infection with parvovirus should be sought.

Haemolysis can occur in sickle cell disorders, and a drop in Hb with a positive haemolytic screen can be caused by a transfusion antibody reaction and worryingly can result in *hyperhaemolysis*, where the antibody response can destroy the patient's native red cells and not just the transfused cells.

This case describes acute chest crisis, and the management is oxygen, intravenous (IV) fluids, pain relief, chest physiotherapy, incentive spirometry and antibiotics. The management is designed to rapidly treat the triggers and prevent further red cell sickling. Blood transfusion or exchange transfusions should be considered early in the hypoxic patient with sickle-negative, Rh and Kell-matched packed red cells. A previous history of red cell antibodies should be sought and appropriate antibody-negative red cells given if applicable.

Future prophylaxis includes a seasonal influenza vaccine, pneumococcal vaccination and offering penicillin V prophylaxis to asplenic patients.

Hydroxycarbamide can be recommended to prevent acute coronary syndrome (ACS).

Consider chronic red cell transfusions if hydroxycarbamide therapy is not effective.

In children, consider a bone marrow transplant if hydroxycarbamide therapy is not effective.

Case 6

A 54-year-old man attends his general practitioner with lethargy and daytime somnolence for 1 year. He has high cholesterol, hypertension and is a non-smoker.

On examination, he has a ruddy facial appearance. O_2 Sats 99% BA, neck collar 18in, weight 120kg, height 5ft 10in.

Hb 180g/L   (130–175)
Hct 0.54   (0.41–0.5)
WCC 9 × 10⁹/L   (4–11)
ANC 7 × 10⁹/L   (2–7.5)
Platelets 320 × 10⁹/L (150–400)

What is the likely cause of the polycythaemia?

a) Chronic lung disease
b) Obstructive sleep apnoea
c) Polycythaemia vera (PV)
d) Dehydration
e) Diuretics

ANSWER CASE 6

Answer: b

Polycythaemia is an increase in the absolute red blood cell mass in the body. In practice, this is reflected by an increase in haemoglobin or haematocrit over the matched age/sex ranges for the patient.

Secondary polycythaemia is more common and can be the result of hypoxic conditions like lung disease, smoking, obstructive sleep apnoea and infrequently the result of exogenous EPO secretion from tumours like red cell counts (RCCs). A mild apparent polycythaemia can be the result of reduced plasma from dehydration or diuretics.

In primary polycythaemia, the bone marrow is overproducing red cells and is labelled as a cancer. The JAK2V617F mutation can be found in over 95% of cases and an exon 12 mutation in some remaining patients.

When the JAK2 mutation is not found, a secondary cause should be sought. A high EPO level would require imaging to look for a tumour-like cerebellar haemangioblastoma, pheochromocytoma, meningioma or a parathyroid tumour.

Polycythaemia vera (PV) can present with arterial or venous occlusive events, or asymptomatic patients can be identified through a full blood count.

Patients with PRV are venesected to a haematocrit <0.45. Aspirin has been demonstrated to reduce thrombotic events.

Cytoreductive therapy with hydroxycarbamide can be considered for selected patients or those not tolerating venesection.

Case 7

A 16-year-old was admitted with cough, sputum and increasing breathlessness. A past medical history of well controlled asthma and coeliacs was noted.

On examination:

RR 24, O_2 Sats 94% on 2 litres (2L) of oxygen
HR 96BPM, BP 124/78mmHg
Auscultation: Crepitations in the right mid zone

Bloods:

CRP 68mg/L   (<5)
WCC 12 × 10⁹/L   (4–11)
Hb 120g/L   (120–175)
Platelets 254 × 10⁹/L (150–400)
Blood film: Neutrophil toxic granulation and vacuolation, occasional Howell–Jolly bodies seen

What is the most appropriate long-term management?

a) No action
b) Long-term steroid-based inhaler to reduce the risk of subsequent infections
c) Longer-term antibiotics with twice-daily salbutamol
d) Patient has dysfunctional spleen and should be managed as asplenic
e) Refer for lung function tests and assess reversibility studies to determine appropriate asthma intervention

ANSWER CASE 7

Answer: d

Patients with an absent or dysfunctional spleen need education regarding the risk of overwhelming infection and the risks of overseas travel, in particular, unusual infections and malaria.

Vaccinations, including pneumococcal, haemophilus influenza type B, meningococcal B, C and yearly influenza, are important.

Patients are encouraged to wear an alert bracelet and carry warning cards for their wallet or purse.

Lifelong prophylactic antibiotics using oral penicillins or macrolides are recommended depending on local pneumococcal resistant patterns.

Causes of dysfunctional or absent spleen:

- Sickle cell disease
- Coeliacs
- Traumatic
- Chronic graft-verse-host disease
- Splenic irradiation

Howell–Jolly bodies are remnants of DNA within red cells and are usually removed by a functioning spleen; therefore, their presence in the circulation indicates a dysfunctional spleen.

Case 8

A 6-year-old male child presents with a swollen knee after minor trauma.

Activated partial thromboplastin time (APTT) 42 seconds   (27–32)
Prothrombin time (PT) 13.2 seconds   (11.7–17.3)
Fibrinogen (FIB) 2.1g/L   (1.5–4.5)

What is the most likely cause?

a) Factor II deficiency
b) Factor VIII deficiency
c) Factor VII deficiency
d) Factor X deficiency
e) Factor XIII deficiency

ANSWER CASE 8

Answer: b

Haemostasis is a highly organised series of events designed to stop blood loss. It involves platelets, procoagulant factors and the vessel wall for the formation of clots. Fibrinolysis is concurrent to ensure the thrombus is confined to the site of injury. Natural anticoagulants circulate to counteract procoagulant factors in health.

The coagulation screen is used to screen procoagulant factors only and therefore is not a robust test for haemostasis. When a patient has a bleeding history, it is utilised to look for a factor deficiency up to factor XII. Factor XIII is not within the in vitro coagulation screen, and when a child is born with profound bleeding and a normal coagulation screen, a separate FXIII assay should be performed. Knowing which factors are confined to the PT and which are confined to the APTT allows the clinician to narrow down the likely factor deficiency. This then allows individual factors to be measured to confirm the diagnosis. This case has a normal PT; therefore, factor VII is normal, and the common factors to the PT and APTT (II, V and X) are at haemostatic levels. An isolated prolonged APTT suspicion is raised for haemophilia A (factor VIII deficiency), haemophilia B (factor IX deficiency), haemophilia C (factor XI deficiency) or factor XII deficiency. Factor XII deficiency is unlikely, as it is not associated with a significant bleeding disposition (see Figure 8.1).

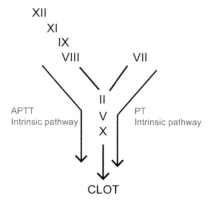

FIGURE 8.1 Procoagulant factors present within the PT and APTT pathway.

Case 9

A 14-year-old attends with severe menorrhagia since menarche last year. She has previously suffered recurrent epistaxis and required a blood transfusion and multiple iron infusions. Her father has a bleeding disorder diagnosed after a minor operation.

Bloods:

Hb 96g/L   (130–175)
MCV 63fL   (80–96)
WCC 9.4 × 10⁹/L   (4–11)
Platelets 235 × 10⁹/L (150–400)
APTT 42secs   (27–32)
PT 13.2secs   (11.7–17.3)
FIB 2.1g/L   (1.5–4.5)

What is the next most appropriate investigation?

a) vWF activity and antigen
b) Factor IV assay
c) Platelet function analyser 100
d) Factor VII assay
e) Factor XII assay

ANSWER CASE 9

Answer: a

von Willebrand factor (vWF) is a polypeptide synthesised in the endothelial cells and megakaryocytes. It is effective at promoting the adhesion and aggregation of platelets, meaning it is essential for primary haemostasis. Interestingly, it is a carrier protein for factor VIII.

Von Willebrand's disease is a bleeding disorder with different types and severities. Most patients present as young adults, and this case is not an unusual presentation. Other presentations include post-partum haemorrhage, bleeding after surgery, dental extractions or cuts, bruising and epistaxis.

The most common type of vWD is type 1, which is a partial quantitative deficiency of vWF. Its mode of inheritance is autosomal dominant. If 1 parent is affected, then there is a 50% chance a son or daughter will have vWD.

The mode of inheritance is a useful discriminator between vWD and haemophilia. vWD can affect males and females given its autosomal mode of inheritance. Haemophilia A and haemophilia B are inherited in an X-linked recessive pattern. The genes are located on the X chromosome. As males only have 1 X chromosome, an inherited gene on this chromosome will give them the disease. Females, because they have 2 X chromosomes, are statistically likely to have at least 1 normal X chromosome, so they will not have the disease but will carry the gene. Typically, with haemophilia A and B in the family pedigree, the males will have a bleeding predisposition, their mothers will be carriers and the maternal father (grandfather) would have been affected. Therefore, haemophilia passes through the maternal lines (see Figure 9.1).

A father with haemophilia passes his only X chromosome to his daughter, and therefore, they will all be carriers (heterozygous). A father passes his Y chromosome to his sons, and therefore, they will not be affected.

Haemophilla Pedigree

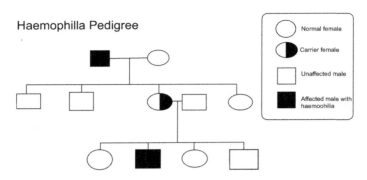

FIGURE 9.1 Typical pedigree demonstrating the inheritance pattern of haemophilia A.

Case 10

A patient with a new diagnosis of acute promyelocytic leukaemia (APL) develops sudden-onset pleuritic chest pain. All-trans-retinoic acid (ATRA) and cytoreductive chemotherapy for the acute leukaemia have already started. There is no evidence of active bleeding, and a computed tomography pulmonary angiogram (CTPA) demonstrates extensive pulmonary emboli.

Bloods:

Hb 84g/L	(130–175)
WCC 34 × 10⁹/L	(4–11)
Blasts 12 × 10⁹/L	
Promyelocytes 16 × 10⁹/L	
Myelocytes 3 × 10⁹/L	
Neutrophils 1 × 10⁹/L	(2–7.5)
Platelets 15 × 10⁹/L	(150–400)
PT 45secs	(11.7–17.3)
APTT 63secs	(27–32)
FIB 0.7g/L	(1.5–4.5)
D-dimer >5000ng/mL	<250ng/mL

What is the most appropriate management?

a) Platelets
b) Fresh frozen plasma (FFP)
c) Cryofibrinogen
d) Unfractionated heparin infusion
e) Low-molecular-weight heparin

ANSWER CASE 10

Answer: d

The combination of a prolonged PT/APTT, low fibrinogen and low platelets with high D-dimer suggests disseminated intravascular coagulation (DIC). DIC is characterised by the activation of coagulation factors and the deposition of fibrin in the microvasculature. In acute DIC, the coagulation factors and platelets are being consumed by thrombi. As control of haemostasis is erratic, the patients may clot, bleed or a mixture.

DIC is not the primary diagnosis, and therefore, the cause must be identified quickly and managed accordingly.

Causes include:

- Infections: Gram positive or negative, EBV, CMV, TB, Fungi and parasites
- Malignancy, especially if disseminated
- Obstetric: Placental abruption, preeclampsia, amniotic fluid emboli
- Extensive trauma, burns or surgery
- Transfusion reaction (mismatched ABO)

Treatment:

Treat the underlying cause/trigger. In this case, the DIC is triggered by APL, and treatment for this has been started.

Next, assess if the patient is bleeding or at a high risk of bleeding or clotting.

If bleeding, platelets can be given via platelet transfusions to increase the platelet count. FFP is used to maintain the PT/APTT within 1.5 upper limit of the normal ULN, and cryoprecipitate or fibrinogen concentrate is used to increase the fibrinogen.

In the situation when a patient is having a clot like this case, then anticoagulation is required. The sensible choice is the drug with the shortest half-life and an antidote, as the patient remains a high risk for a bleed.

Case 11

A previously well 45-year-old female attends after a witnessed seizure. She has noticed over the last few days increased tiredness, and her friends have commented on her yellowing sclera.

Bloods:

Hb 85g/L	(130–175)
Blood film: Schistocytes with a true thrombocytopenia	
WCC 4.5 × 10⁹/L	(4–11)
Platelets 54 × 10⁹/L	(150–400)
Bilirubin 75μmol/L	(<17)
Crea 400μmol/L	(60–120)
Direct bilirubin 10μmol/L	
GFR 13mL/min/1.73m²	(>60)
GGT 64IU/L	(10–40)
Troponin 250ng/L	(<14)
ALP 155IU/L	(25–115)
D-dimer 300ng/mL	(<250)
AST 90IU/L	(10–40)
PT 14secs	(11.7–17.3)
ALT 65IU/L	(10–50)
APTT 31secs	(27–32)
FIB 2g/L	(1.5–4.5)

Pregnancy test negative

What is the likely diagnosis?

a) DIC
b) Haemolysis, elevated liver enzymes, low platelets (HELLP)
c) Metastatic cancer
d) Thrombotic thrombocytopenia purpura (TTP)
e) Haemolytic uraemic syndrome (HUS)

DOI: 10.1201/9781003501190-13

ANSWER CASE 11

Answer: d

Schistocytes are red cell fragments and can be a worrying sign when seen in the presence of a thrombocytopenia. The term used to describe this is microangiopathic haemolytic anaemia (MAHA) with thrombocytopenia. Causes of this can include:

- DIC
- HELLP, preeclampsia, eclampsia
- HUS
- Atypical HUS (aHUS)
- TTP
- Others: Medications and rare reports with COVID-19

DIC can be diagnosed from a prolonged PT/APTT, low fibrinogen and low platelets.

Pregnancy-associated HELLP can progress to pre-eclampsia or eclampsia, and the management is delivery of the child.

Haemolytic uraemic syndrome (HUS) is typically a diarrhoeal illness triggered by *E. coli* 0157 followed by a microangiopathic haemolytic anaemia (MAHA) and isolated kidney injury.

Atypical HUS is without the diarrhoeal illness but the presence of acute kidney injury with the MAHA and thrombocytopenia.

Cases of MAHA and thrombocytopenia have been reported with certain cancers, drugs and a COVID-related trigger.

Information has been provided to exclude the differentials of DIC and pregnancy-related complications. The organ damage is not isolated to the kidneys, therefore making HUS/aHUS less likely. Evidence of thrombus formation with the elevated D-dimer and organ damage with the liver, kidneys and heart all suggest a catastrophic systemic disease. Based on the information provided, this is a case of TTP which has a poor prognosis when undiagnosed.

Immediate plasma exchange is justified while awaiting for the confirmatory ADAMTS13 assay results.

Case 12

A 16-year-old attends with jaundice and tiredness over the past few weeks. On further questioning, his mother informs you he had prolonged jaundice at birth but no other health concerns. Family history reveals his father died in an accident at age 30, but his father's only bother had both his spleen and gallbladder removed at age 20.

Hb 86g/L   (130–175)
WCC 7.8 × 10⁹/L   (4–11)
Platelets 250 × 10⁹/L   (150–400)
LDH 400IU/L   (70–250)
Reticulocytes 5.6%   (1–2%)
Blood film: Spherocytes, polychromasia
Haptoglobin: Absent
DAT/Coombs: Negative

What is the likely diagnosis?

a) Hereditary spherocytosis
b) Acquired warm autoimmune haemolytic anaemia
c) Zieve's
d) Glucose-6-phosphate dehydrogenase (G6PD) deficiency
e) Pyruvate kinase (PK) deficiency

ANSWER CASE 12

Answer: a

The current age of the patient and prolonged jaundice at birth would be suspicious of an inherited condition. The increase in indirect bilirubin, reticulocytes, LDH and absent haptoglobin suggests haemolysis.

The blood film shows spherocytes, and direct antibody test (DAT) is negative, therefore going against an immune trigger. The most likely diagnosis is hereditary spherocytosis.

A family history of HS and the presence of spherocytic DAT negative haemolysis is enough to make a diagnosis of HS. However as 25% of patients presence without a family history then Eosin-5-malemide (EMA) binding has a high predictive value. Hereditary spherocytosis results from a deficiency in one or more membrane proteins resulting in the inability to maintain their normal biconcave shape. The most common protein membrane defect in HS is due to Ankyrin deficiency and to a lesser degree spectrin, band 3 and protein 4.2. Another interesting red cell membrance disorder is Hereditary elliptocytosis (HE). In HE, the same clinical presentation can be expected but instead of spherocytes on the blood film it will have elliptocytes. This autosomal dominant disorder is mostly caused by a defect in the spectrin protein.

If the DAT was positive for IgG, then the pattern could be in keeping with warm autoimmune haemolytic anaemia.

There is no history of alcohol, making Zieve's unlikely. Both G6PD and PK deficiency are inherited causes of haemolysis, but different morphology would be expected on the blood film. G6PD deficiency predisposes haemoglobin to oxidative damage. The haemoglobin denatures and clumps as a Heinz body to the periphery of the cell. The spleen macrophage engulfs this, resulting in a 'bite cell'. Therefore, the blood film should reveal bite cells as the cause for haemolysis. G6PD deficiency is inherited in an X-linked recessive manner and therefore more common in males. Triggers include many drugs, viruses, eating fava beans and moth balls.

Testing to confirm diagnosis needs to wait until the acute haemolytic episode has resolved. During a crisis, the compensatory reticulocytosis can result in false normal G6PD levels as reticulocytes carry more enzyme.

PK deficiency is another rare inherited cause of haemolysis, but this time, the red cells would have a prickle appearance (echinocytes) on the blood film.

Case 13

A well 6-year-old attends with a petechial rash on their lower legs. There is no neck stiffness or pyrexia.

Hb 123g/L   (120–175)
WCC 6.5 × 10⁹/L   (4–11)
Platelets 4 × 10⁹/L   (150–400)
Blood film: No platelet clumps
Coagulation screen: Normal
Urinalysis: NAD

What is the most likely diagnosis?

a) ITP
b) TTP
c) DIC
d) Meningitis
e) Vasculitis

ANSWER CASE 13

Answer: a

Bruising is bleeding within the skin and is classified by the size. The size gives us a clue to the underlying aetiology.

Petechiae are small and no more than a few millimetres. They are non-blanching and caused by capillary leak. Causes can include meningitis (but this child is too well), as well as other infections like CMV, EBV and streptococcus. There are no symptoms to suggest infection.

Vasculitis can present with a similar rash and result in organ damage. There are no systemic symptoms with this case and no evidence of renal damage, making vasculitis and TTP less likely with the information provided. DIC is excluded by a normal coagulation screen.

Immune thrombocytopenia purpura (ITP) is the most likely diagnosis and in children this young may not require any treatment unless overt bleeding is present. It can spontaneously resolve in children. In adults, ITP is treated with steroids or IV immunoglobins in the acute situation. Other medications include thrombopoietin (TPO) agonists and anti-CD20 monoclonal antibodies. In elderly patients presenting with low platelets, it is more difficult to distinguish between ITP and myelodysplasia (MDS).

Case 14

An 80-year-old nursing home resident attends the ED with new-onset right hemiparesis. Brain CT demonstrates an intracranial haemorrhage. INR is 3.5.

What is the most appropriate next step?

a) Vitamin K
b) FFP
c) Fibrinogen concentrate
d) Vitamin K plus prothrombin complex concentrate (PCC)
e) PCC

DOI: 10.1201/9781003501190-16

ANSWER CASE 14

Answer: d

This case tests your knowledge on warfarin reversal. Although we are not informed that this patient is on warfarin, an INR has been checked and therefore makes this likely. The INR is a standardised PT used to monitor warfarin. PT can vary based on the analyser and reagent used to measure them. Laboratories apply a correction to their PT to give an international normalised ratio (INR), allowing patients on warfarin the ability to get an INR check in any laboratory across all hospitals.

$$INR = (tested\ PT\ /\ normal\ PT)^{ISI}$$

The ISI stands for International Sensitivity Index and standardises the difference between PT assays.

Warfarin competitively inhibits VKORC1 vitamin K epoxide reductase complex 1, which is essential for activating vitamin K for vitamin K-dependent procoagulant factors FII, VII, IX and X and anticoagulants protein C, S and Z.

When warfarinising patients with acute venous thromboembolism (VTE), they require bridging with low-molecular-weight heparin (LMWH), as during initial warfarinisation, there is a drop in natural anticoagulation prior to procoagulants, initially making a thrombotic patient even more thrombotic.

The decision to reverse warfarin, and how to, depends on the clinical situation.

In this case it is a life-threatening bleed, and therefore, immediate reversal is required with PCC; remember that factor II in PCC degrades at 6 hours, much shorter than the half-life of warfarin (20–60 hours). Vitamin K must be given at the same time as PCC, and the effect of Vitamin K occurs at 6 hours as the PCC loses effect.

If the INR is 5.0–8.0 with no bleeding, withhold a couple of doses warfarin.

If the INR is 5.0–8.0 with minor bleeding, stop warfarin and give vitamin K.

If the INR is >8.0 with mild bleeding or no bleeding, stop warfarin and give vitamin K, as the patient is at high risk of major bleeding.

Case 15

A 65-year-old with non-valvular AF is currently on apixaban 5mg BD. His last dose of medication was 2 hours ago. He was admitted with a 1-hour history of tiredness and melaena.

On examination:

HR 150BPM
BP 75/30mmHg
Sats 94% on breathing air
RR 22

What is the most suitable reversal agent?

a) FFP
b) PCC
c) Idarucizumab
d) Andexanet alpha
e) Vitamin K

DOI: 10.1201/9781003501190-17

Answer: d

Anticoagulation medications are used widely and have different modes of action on the coagulation cascade. Apixaban's mode of action is direct inhibition of activated Factor X (FXa). Their elimination depends on the drug half-life and organ reserve depending on how the drug is metabolised.

In many cases of minor bleeding, simple, non-pharmacological measures are all that's required while awaiting natural clearance of the anticoagulant.

In emergency cases when pharmacological intervention is required, there are licensed drugs:

Idarucimab is licensed for the rapid reversal of dabigatran in a life-threatening bleed or emergency surgery that cannot wait.

Andexanet alfa is licensed for the reversal of apixaban or rivaroxaban in a life-threatening GI bleed.

PCC is used in the emergency reversal of warfarin in a life-threatening bleed.

FFP is not used a reversal for direct oral anticoagulants but is used in a bleed to replace factors if there is a global deficiency, for example, in a massive haemorrhage or liver disease.

Vitamin K in isolation is very useful to reverse the effects of warfarin but takes 6 hours and is therefore used for haemostatic patients that can wait.

As vitamin K decreases, the levels of activated factors II, VII, IX and X will decrease, causing prolongation of both the PT and APTT.

Although we do not use the coagulation screen to assess if a patient is on a DOAC or use it to assess its effect on anticoagulation, it is important to know its effect in case there is dual pathology, like a combined vitamin K deficiency or acquired haemophilia.

Dabigatran increases the TT, while apixaban, edoxaban and rivaroxaban have no effect.

Apixaban has little to no effect on APTT, while edoxaban, rivaroxaban and dabigatran can have a mild to moderate effect.

Slight rises in PT can be seen with dabigatran, rivaroxaban, apixaban and edoxaban.

Levels of apixaban, edoxaban or rivaroxaban are not generally required but can be measured with a drug-specific anti-Xa level.

Warfarin does need to be monitored with an INR, and dietary education is required due to the effects of vitamin K-containing foods. Also, care needs to be taken when prescribing drugs that interfere with cytochrome P450. Kidney function is not relevant when prescribing warfarin. Another anticoagulant for which patients need dietary advice is 15mg and 20mg of rivaroxaban, as patients need to take these medications with food to allow absorption.

The anti-Xa inhibitors like LMWH, oral apixaban, edoxaban and rivaroxaban have their onset within a few hours, while warfarin takes days.

Only a good understanding of an anticoagulant's mode of action, metabolism and excretion allows the physician to prescribe the most suitable drug to a patient taking their co-morbidities into account.

Case 16

A 45-year-old man from Magherafelt, Northern Ireland, presents with arthralgia and general tiredness. He was diagnosed with diabetes 2 years ago.

On examination, he has a bronze complexion.

His FBC is normal
Ferritin 2543µg/L   (30–400)
Sats 70%
CRP <5mg/L

What genetic pattern would most commonly explain these findings?

a) Homozygous c282y
b) Heterozygous for c282y
c) Homozygous for H63D
d) Heterozygous for H63D
e) *SLC40A1* (2q32) mutation

DOI: 10.1201/9781003501190-18

ANSWER CASE 16

Answer: a

Genetic haemochromatosis (GH) is one of the most common genetic conditions to affect Northern Europeans. In normal health, when iron stores are adequate, the body reduces the absorption of iron in the small bowel. In GH, the iron absorption continues, and as the body cannot excrete iron adequately, this leads to accumulation. In severe cases, the accumulation of iron in organs causes damage. Excess iron in the liver can result in cirrhosis and increase the risk of hepatic cellular carcinoma. Patients with a ferritin level >1000µg/L require surveillance with ultrasound and alpha fetoprotein measurements every 6 months. Iron deposition in the joints can cause arthritis, the 2nd and 3rd metacarpophalangeal joints being the typical site. Deposition in the pancreas can result in diabetes. Iron deposition can occur in the heart, resulting in conduction issues or cardiomyopathy, but this is more common with transfusion-associated iron overload than GH.

If a patient has elevated ferritin and Sats, they should get a genetic *HFE* gene analysis. The gene is located on chromosome 6 near the HLA-A location. It is inherited as autosomal recessive, and therefore 2 copies are required for the condition. C282Y mutation of the *HFE* gene is more common in Northern Europeans than H63D.

Treatment is venesection weekly to get the ferritin below 20–30µg/L then long-term venesections to maintain the serum ferritin (SF) <50µg/L. If the patient had no evidence of cirrhosis, they may be suitable for long-term blood donations.

Case 17

A 37-year-old para 4 presents in her 2nd trimester with left-sided leg swelling. It was first noticed 2 days ago and is becoming increasingly uncomfortable. Ultrasound confirms extensive thrombosis extending into the common femoral vein.

BMI 32 pre-pregnancy

On examination, she has a left swollen, tender leg with varicose veins noted bilaterally.

What is the most appropriate treatment option?

a) Warfarin
b) Apixaban
c) Dabigatran
d) Low-molecular-weight heparin
e) Rivaroxaban

ANSWER CASE 17

Answer: d

Pregnancy is associated with a 10-fold increased risk of venous thrombo-embolism compared to the non-pregnant state. The risk continues to 6 weeks post-partum.

UK guidelines RCOG in 2015 recommend a VTE risk assessment to identify at-risk woman for consideration of prophylactic treatment.

Risk factors include age >35, obesity, parity ≥3, previous VTE and known thrombophilia, as well as other obstetric and transient risk factors.

This case, with the patient's age >35, obesity, parity ≥3 and varicose veins has 4 risk factors and should have been considered for thromboprophylaxis from 1st trimester.

LMWH is the drug of choice for antenatal and postnatal thromboprophylaxis. Heparins have a large molecular weight and do not cross the placenta or cross into breast milk in the postnatal stage.

DOACs should not be taken during pregnancy, and small amounts can be detected in breast milk.

Warfarin is not recommended, as it can cause birth defects. Warfarin can be used during breast feeding; the small amounts detected are unlikely to have any side effects on the baby.

Case 18

A 65-year-old man presents with sudden-onset pleuritic pain on the right side of his chest.

He was previously well with no past medical history of cancer, heart failure or lung disease.

On examination:

HR 110BPM
BP 90/70
RR 32
T°C 36.7

What is the most useful diagnostic test for the likely diagnosis?

a) 12 lead ECG
b) Transoesophageal echocardiography
c) CT pulmonary angiography
d) Isotope lung scan
e) Blood D-dimer

DOI: 10.1201/9781003501190-20

Answer: c
Pulmonary embolism is when 1 or more emboli travel to the pulmonary arterial system. The most common source is a DVT from the lower limbs.

Risk factors for a PE include:

- DVT
- Cancer
- Recent surgery
- Immobilisation
- Pregnancy and up to 6 weeks post-partum
- Significant immobility like hospitalisation
- Age >60
- Long-haul flights
- cOCP/HRT
- Known thrombophilia

A 2-level PE Wells score should be used to estimate the risk of PE. If >4, then a computed tomography pulmonary angiogram (CTPA) should be performed. If it cannot be immediately performed, then the patient should start therapeutic anticoagulation until offered.

If the Wells score is ≤4, then a D-dimer is performed and results made available within 4 hours. If the D-dimer is negative, another diagnosis should be looked for, and if the D-dimer is positive, then a CTPA should be arranged.

Therapeutic anticoagulation should continue for 3 months and the patient provided with an anticoagulation alert card. The patient should receive written and verbal information on the anticoagulant.

Long-term prophylaxis should be offered after the 3 months of therapeutic anticoagulation if the patient has had an unprovoked VTE or an ongoing risk factor like active cancer. The risk for long-term anticoagulation should be weighed up against the patient's bleeding risk and again the patient should be counselled regarding this risk/benefit.

Case 19

A 54-year-old female presents with a pale, painful right foot.

She has never been to hospital apart from when she had three miscarriages.

On examination, the dorsalis pedis pulse is absent, and her toes look necrotic.

Bloods:

Hb 145g/L   (120–175)
WCC 5.6 × 10⁹/L   (4–11)
Platelets 43 × 10⁹/L (150–400)

What blood test would help confirm the underlying diagnosis?

a) B12 and folate
b) JAK2V617F mutation
c) Lupus anticoagulant
d) Homocysteine level
e) dsDNA

Answer: c

Arterial thrombus is a blood clot in an artery. This has a different pathophysiology from venous clots.

Arterial clots include myocardial infarctions, cerebrovascular accidents, transient ischaemic attacks and peripheral artery diseases.

These conditions are emergencies because the tissue distal to the clot becomes ischaemic.

Risk factors for atherosclerosis include:

- Age
- Smoking
- Reduced exercise
- Obesity
- Alcohol
- Hypertension, hypercholesterolaemia, diabetes
- Family history
- Ethnic origin: Asian, African or African-Caribbean

Despite atherosclerosis risk factors, arterial clots can happen in otherwise healthy vasculature. If this occurs, the patient needs investigated for rarer causes like:

- Antiphospholipid syndrome: test with anticardiolipin antibody, β2 glycoprotein and lupus anticoagulant
- Myeloproliferative cause: screen with JAK2V617F mutation analysis
- Homocysteine
- Paroxysmal nocturnal haemoglobinuria (PNH) screen

In patients with arterial clots or unprovoked venous clots in unusual places, this should raise suspicion of an underlying condition like those described.

section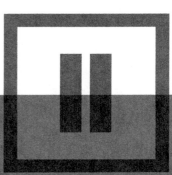

Transfusion Medicine

Case 20

A 65-year-old tree surgeon received trauma to his arm damaging his brachial artery. On arrival to the emergency department, the heart rate was 140BPM and systolic BP 80mmHg despite 2 litres of crystalloid. Tranexamic acid bolus of 1g was administered followed by an infusion.

No blood group was available on admission; therefore, 6 units of group O packed red cells and 4 units of FFP had been transfused. Post-resuscitation, the patients bleeding had stopped, HR was 80BPM and systolic BP 110mmHg.

The repeat coagulation screen post-resuscitation:

PT 17secs   (27–32)
APTT 24secs   (11.7–17.3)
FIB 0.8g/L   (1.5–4.5)

What is the next most appropriate step?

a) Transfuse platelets
b) Transfuse FFP 15–20mL/kg
c) Give a further bolus of tranexamic acid
d) Cryofibrinogen
e) PCC

ANSWER CASE 20

Answer: d

There are numerous definitions of major haemorrhage based on the quantity of blood loss; however, the current trend is towards the clinical context and the physiological response to bleeding. For example, HR >110 +/− SBP <90

Frontline clinical staff are trained to recognise major blood loss early and activate the local major haemorrhage protocol. Hospitals have a strategy to ensure that emergency group O RhD-, K-negative is available for females of childbearing potential or Group O + for a male until their exact blood group is known.

If major bleeding is ongoing and no TEG or coagulation screen is available to guide plasma product use, then it is recommended to use FFP in at least a 1:2 ratio with units of packed red cells being transfused.

When coagulation screen results are available:

FFP 15–20mL/kg is to be administered to maintain the PT ratio at <1.5 times the upper limit of normal (ULN).

Fibrinogen supplementation (cryoprecipitate or fibrinogen concentrate) should be given if fibrinogen concentrations fall below 1.5g/L (non-pregnant women). Thrombocytopenia is a late effect in a major haemorrhage at is not expected until 1.5 blood volumes are lost. Platelet transfusions should be used to maintain platelet counts at >50 × 10^9/L.

Tranexamic acid is recommended for patients with presentations of major bleeding due to trauma but not in gastrointestinal bleeding.

Case 21

A 38-year-old female successfully delivered twins. Four hours post-delivery, vaginal blood loss was estimated at 1000mL.

IV fluids, tranexamic acid and numerous packed red cells were transfused. Ultrasound (US) revealed no retained products, and bleeding had reduced but was still ongoing.

Blood results return:

Hb 92g/L	(130–175)
WCC 9 × 10⁹/L	(4–11)
Platelets 176 × 10⁹/L	(150–400)
PT 16secs	(11.7–17.3)
APTT 32secs	(27–32)
FIB 1.8g/L	(1.5–4.5)

What product should be considered?

a) Packed red cells
b) Platelets
c) FFP
d) Fibrinogen concentrate
e) PCC

ANSWER CASE 21

Answer: d

Post-partum haemorrhage (PPH) is a serious, life-threatening condition that usually happens within 24 hours after giving birth but can occur up to 12 weeks. Under normal circumstances post-delivery, the uterus contacts, which helps compress blood vessels that were in the area the placenta was attached.

It can happen to 1–5% of women, but there are risk factors including placenta abruption, placenta previa, multiple pregnancies, traumatic deliveries and pre-existing fibroids.

Primary PPH is the loss of >500mL of blood within 24 hours of delivery; >1000mL is classified as major. Secondary PPH is bleeding from 24 hours to 12 weeks after birth.

The same recommendations with tranexamic acid, packed red cells (PRCs) and FFP as per the major haemorrhage protocol should be used. However, fibrinogen replacement should occur if fibrinogen levels are <2.0g/L.

Case 22

An 80-year-old man admitted last week with a non-ST-elevation
myocardial infarction (NSTEMI) received a unit of packed red cells
5 hours ago for a haemoglobin of 70g/L.

He developed dyspnoea and desaturated to 89% BA.

On examination, he had an increased jugular venous pressure (JVP)
and bilateral crepitations on auscultation.

What is the likely cause of the dyspnoea?

a) Transfusion-related acute lung injury (TRALI)
b) Transfusion-associated circulatory overload (TACO)
c) Hospital-acquired pneumonia
d) Acute haemolytic transfusion reaction
e) Febrile non-haemolytic transfusion reaction

ANSWER CASE 22

Answer: b

TACO is pulmonary oedema within 6 hours of a blood transfusion. It is the most common cause of transfusion-related death in developed countries.

The signs/symptoms are similar to heart failure with pulmonary creps, increase JVP, hypertension, tachycardia and evidence of a positive fluid balance.

The predisposing factors for getting TACO are renal failure, known heart failure, low albumin, positive fluid balance and low body weight.

Treatment is oxygen with a diuretic and to prevent further events. Premedication with a diuretic can be used with a slow transfusion over 3hr 30min.

A transfused unit of blood in an average-weight patient (70–80kg) should increase haemoglobin by 10g/L. If the body weight is less, a unit would increase Hb further, and patients can be at increased risk of TACO. In those patients with low body weight/frailty, blood can be prescribed at 4mL/kg (paediatric practice).

Case 23

An 18-year-old male is in a road traffic collision. His femoral vasculature was compromised, and given the profuse blood loss, the massive blood transfusion protocol was activated in the emergency department.

During resuscitation, he received 8 units of packed red cells, 4 units of FFP and 2 units of platelets.

Within 6 hours of his transfusions, he developed shortness of breath, fever and hypotension.

His chest X-ray showed bilateral infiltrates.

What is the most likely cause of his dyspnoea?

a) TACO
b) TRALI
c) Pneumonia
d) Pneumocystis Jiroveci pneumonia (PJP)
e) Haemolytic transfusion reaction

DOI: 10.1201/9781003501190-26

ANSWER CASE 23

Answer: b

TRALI is characterised by breathlessness and lung infiltrates within 6 hours of a blood transfusion. It is an antibody-mediated condition were the donor antibodies react with the patient's pulmonary endothelium or inflammatory cells.

Treatment is supportive with oxygen and ventilation support if required. Most patients survive with support and recover within 72 hours.

The main differential of TRALI is TACO, as both patients present with breathlessness, decreased oxygen saturation and pulmonary infiltrates. The important difference is that in TRALI, the JVP should be lower normal, while in TACO, the JVP is elevated. In TRALI, the temperature is often elevated, and the neutrophils/monocytes fall initially, but then the neutrophils increase. With TACO, the blood counts are non-specific, and the temperature is normal.

As the blood pressure drops in TRALI, fluid challenges can help and diuretics can worsen the scenario; with TACO, the reverse is true.

In the UK, transfusion reactions are investigated by the haemovigilance team. This is a systematic review of adverse reactions and adverse events related to transfusion with the aim of improving safety. These events are investigated by the hospital transfusion team (HTT) and reviewed by the hospital transfusion committee HTC and if deemed appropriated are reported to Serious Hazards of Transfusion (SHOT) and the Medicines and Healthcare Products Regulatory Agency (MHRA).

Case 24

A 65-year-old patient on long-term blood product support was receiving a unit of packed red cells. Thirty minutes into the transfusion, the temperature was recorded at 38.2°C. The baseline temperature was 37.5°C. The patient felt well, with no pain at the transfusion site and no bone pain. The patient was treated with an anti-pyretic to good effect, and the transfusion temporarily slowed down. The transfusion continued uneventfully, and the patient remained well in the days after.

What is the likely classification of this transfusion reaction?

a) TACO
b) TRALI
c) Febrile non-haemolytic transfusion reaction (FNHTR)
d) Delayed haemolytic transfusion reaction (DHTR)
e) Post-transfusion purpura

ANSWER CASE 24

Answer: c

FNHTR is now less common since blood products have been leucodepleted. It is more common in patients who have undergone multiple transfusions.

Mild temperatures can be treated with anti-pyretics, and the transfusion can be temporarily slowed down or stopped. The patients are observed closely for signs of a more severe ATR like unstable observations, pain at the infusion site, bone pain or any anaphylactic signs. In the majority of patients with FNHTR, the temperature settles quickly, and the rest of the transfusion remains uneventful. It is important to note the product needs to be transfused within its cold-chain life.

Case 25

A 45-year-old patient with known severe aplastic anaemia has recently moved country and attended his new haematology unit for a unit of packed red cells.

Less than 1 minute into transfusion, he developed severe pain at the site of the venous access, hypotension, tachycardia, rigors and nausea.

What is the most appropriate immediate action?

a) Oxygen
b) IV fluids
c) Stop the transfusion
d) Assess A, B, C
e) Report immediately to SHOT

ANSWER CASE 25

Answer: c

Acute transfusion reactions (ATRs) present within 24 hours of a transfusion and include:

- TACO
- TRALI
- Acute haemolytic transfusion reactions
- FNHTR
- Bacterial contamination of the unit
- Allergic reactions

Allergic reactions can vary from urticaria to full anaphylaxis. Consider measuring serial mast cell tryptase to confirm diagnoses. Patients should have IgA levels checked, and the Asian population have haptoglobin levels checked. Deficiencies in either can result in an anaphylactic reaction. For IgA deficiency, patients could be transfused from IgA-deficient donors or, if time doesn't allow, wash products.

FNHTR as discussed is usually an isolated pyrexia and provided the temperature is <39°C or not ≥2°C from baseline, transfusion is continued, and generally, these are not reported to the HTT, HTC or SHOT.

The bacterial contamination of products should be considered if the temperature rises to ≥39°C or ≥2°C from baseline. Patients can develop signs/symptoms of sepsis. The product which is most commonly implicated is platelets, and they should be visually inspected for contamination and returned for culture. The patient should also have blood cultures. If the product is found to be the cause, then other products that the donor has donated are removed to prevent other reactions. This adverse event would be reviewed at the HTC.

Both TACO and TRALI are reportable and should be investigated by the HTT/HTC and reported to SHOT/MHRA.

In this case, the immediate symptoms and pain at the access point are very concerning for acute haemolytic transfusion reactions (AHTRs) such as ABO incompatibility.

First, stop the transfusion immediately and maintain venous access. Resuscitation—airway, breathing and circulation should be ongoing.

Full bloods including FBP, renal and liver function, urine for Hb, repeat samples for compatibility testing, direct antiglobulin test, LDH, haptoglobins, coagulation screen and blood cultures should be performed.

The implicated unit must not be discarded and returned. An ABO mismatch is a never event and must be investigated by the HTT and HTC and reported to SHOT/MHRA.

Case 26

A 37-year-old multiparous female suffered a post-partum haemorrhage after the birth of her 3rd child. She received 2 units of packed cells and was discharged several days later. She presented 7 days later with tiredness and a yellow discolouration of her skin and sclera.

Hb 85g/L	(130–175)
WCC 8 × 10^9/L	(4–11)
Platelets 168 × 10^9/L	(150–400)
Total bilirubin 120µmol/L	(<21)
Direct bilirubin 15µmol/L	
LDH 300IU/L	(70–250)
Haptoglobin absent	
Reticulocytes 15%	(1–2)
DAT-positive IgG	

Which antibody is most likely to be implicated?

a) Anti-A
b) Anti-B
c) Anti-D
d) Kidd (Jk)
e) Anti-C

ANSWER CASE 26

Answer: d

This is a case of a delayed haemolytic transfusion reaction (DHTR). This women has likely been alloimmunised during a previous pregnancy. It is also possible to be alloimmunised through previous blood transfusions. These antibodies are likely to be at such a low level that the pre-compatibility antibody screen has not detected them. The transfused blood then contains the corresponding antigen, boosting up the antibody and resulting in haemolysis, typically days later.

Kidd (Jk) antibodies are the most common followed by Rh antibodies. Remember that these reactions are caused by IgG antibodies and not IgM antibodies, which are implicated in ABO mismatch. The ABO mismatch IgM reactions trigger immediate activation of the complement and coagulation cascade and can have fatal results.

With DHTR, the patient is issued an antibody card, and computer records are updated to ensure the patient is not suitable for automated crossmatch.

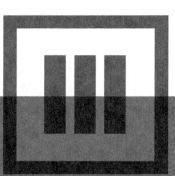

section III

Malignant Haematology

Case 27

A 3-year-old boy presents to the emergency department with weakness, dizziness and difficult breathing. He is having temperatures of 38°C.

Bloods:

Hb 95g/L   (130–175)
WCC 65 × 10⁹/L   (4–11)
Blasts 62 × 10⁹/L
Platelets 80 × 10⁹/L   (150–400)
Chest X-ray demonstrates mediastinal widening.

What is the likely diagnosis?

a) T-acute lymphoblastic leukaemia (T-ALL)
b) B-ALL
c) Hodgkin lymphoma
d) Teratoma
e) Lower respiratory tract infection with sepsis

Answer: a

The bone marrow produces stem cells, whose role is to produce blood cells. Myeloid stem cells go through different stages of maturation with the aim of ultimately making mature neutrophils, red cells and megakaryocytes (platelet production). Mature neutrophils, red cells and platelets then circulate in the blood stream. Lymphoid stem cells go through maturation in the bone marrow to make B lymphocytes, T lymphocytes and natural killer (NK) cells. The immature precursors in normal health stay in the bone marrow. Interestingly, both B and T lymphocytes are produced in the bone marrow, but B lymphocytes mature in the bone marrow and T cells mature in the thymus before entering the peripheral circulation. The thymus is a small organ that lies behind the sternum.

The differential diagnosis of a mediastinal mass is (4Ts) thymoma, T-cell lymphoma or leukaemia, thyroid with retrosternal expansion and teratoma.

During sepsis, the demand for blood cells increases therefore immature precursors can be released, and this is called left shift. With left shift, the cells circulating are close to maturation and mixed with mature cells. Blasts, which are the earliest stage of development, are infrequent. When blasts are present in large numbers without maturation, then this is in keeping with acute leukaemia.

Leukaemia is cancer of the body's blood-forming tissues, and many types exist. Leukaemia usually involves the white blood cells that normally fight infection. Acute leukaemia is when a primitive cell divides uncontrollably and generally loses its ability to mature into its intended cell. Acute lymphoblastic leukaemia is the most common childhood leukaemia and characterised by an excess of lymphoid blasts.

Chemotherapy is the main treatment, and some high-risk individuals require a bone marrow transplant.

Treatment is done in steps, including remission induction, consolidation and then a maintenance phase.

Unfavourable prognosis in ALL includes age <1 or >10 years, male, central nervous system (CNS) as manifested by leukaemic cells in cerebrospinal fluid (CSF) or testicular involvement, hypodiploidy and presence of mutations like t(4;11).

The *BCR-ABL* fusion gene and product resulting from t(9;22), if present, requires the addition of a tyrosine kinase inhibitor to the chemotherapy to offset its poor prognosis. It is interesting that hyperdiploidy is associated with a better prognosis, but overall, the survival in childhood ALL is over 90% at 5 years.

Case 28

A 26-year-old girl presents with tiredness and reduced exercise tolerance over the past 2 weeks. She has developed a cough with pyrexia in the past 48 hours.

Hb 123g/L   (130–175)
WCC 18 × 10⁹/L   (4–11)
Platelets 67 × 10⁹/L   (150–400)
CRP 65mg/L   (<5)

The blood analyser has flagged blasts, and a manual blood film has been reported.
About 25% of nucleated cells are blasts, with occasional Auer rods seen.

What is the unifying diagnosis?

a) Acute lymphoblastic leukaemia
b) Acute myeloid leukaemia
c) Sepsis
d) Bone metastasis of a solid tumour
e) Chronic lymphocytic leukaemia

ANSWER CASE 28

Answer: b

Over 20% blasts in the bone marrow or peripheral blood is diagnostic of acute leukaemia. Sometimes a lower blast count with certain genetic alterations can also confirm AML. The presence of Auer rods tell us they are of myeloid lineage, and therefore, the diagnosis is acute myeloid leukaemia (AML).

Auer rods are azurophilic cytoplasmic inclusions that can resemble needles and are specific to myeloid blast cells.

Patients presenting with acute leukaemia can present with signs/symptoms associated with bone marrow failure like anaemia or bleeding from thrombocytopenia. The excess blasts can result in reduced mature white cells and, therefore, as in this case, present with an active infection.

Case 29

A 19-year-old man presents to the ED with a 2-week history of tiredness. He has noticed extensive petechiae, purpura and areas of ecchymosis. He is haemodynamically stable with no active bleeding or clinical evidence of VTE.

Hb 115g/L   (130–175)
WCC 23 × 10⁹/L   (4–11)
Blasts 15 × 10⁹/L
Promyelocytes 4 × 10⁹/L %
Neutrophils 2 × 10⁹/L
Platelets 8 × 10⁹/L   (150–400)

Blood film: Blasts and frequent promyelocytes. Auer rods seen.

PT 26secs   (11.7–17.3)
APTT 53secs   (27–32)
FIB 0.8g/L   (1.5–4.5)
Genetics: t(15;17)

What immediate treatment does this patient need?

a) All-trans-retinoic acid (ATRA)
b) Arsenic trioxide
c) Idarubicin
d) CT chest, abdomen and pelvis
e) Unfractionated heparin infusion

ANSWER CASE 29

Answer: a

The prolongation in PT and APTT suggest a global deficiency in procoagulant clotting factors. This, combined with low fibrinogen, low platelets and increased D-dimer, raises concern of micro thrombi consumed with platelets and factors. This pattern is in keeping with disseminated intravascular coagulation (DIC).

DIC is triggered by another process, including sepsis, cancers and, in this case, by leukaemia.

The presence of promyelocytes with the blasts is in keeping with a type of acute myeloid leukaemia called acute promyelocytic leukaemia (APL).

This type of leukaemia commonly presents with a patient in DIC and needing urgent treatment before a life-threatening bleed or clot occurs.

The promyelocytes in the disease are what's triggering the DIC, and therefore, all-trans-retinoic acid (ATRA) is given, which results in the promyelocytes maturing beyond this stage. The ATRA should be started as soon as possible, and thereafter, arsenic trioxide or idarubicin is started to reduce the amount of disease. ATRA, especially if there's a delay in chemotherapy, results in a rapid increase in the white cell count, resulting in ATRA syndrome/differentiation syndrome. ATRA syndrome is characterised by fever, peripheral oedema, pulmonary infiltrates, hypotension and acute renal impairment.

APL is caused by t(15;17), PML RARA, and despite its concerning presentation, it carries one of the better long-term prognoses in AML.

Case 30

A 53-year-old lady attends with early satiety. On examination, there is a palpable mass in the left upper quadrant extending to the right iliac fossa. The upper margin is not able to be ascertained, and it is not ballotable. It is dull to percussion and moves with respiration.

Hb 123g/L	(130–175)
WCC 213 × 10⁹/L	(4–11)

Neutrophils 179 × 10⁹/L
Basophils 7 × 10⁹/L
Eosinophils 2 × 10⁹/L
Lymphocytes 3 × 10⁹/L
Myelocytes 10 × 10⁹/L

What genetic mutation is most likely?

a) BCR-ABL t(9;22)
b) JAK2 V617F
c) CALR
d) PML RARA t(15;17)
e) MLL 11q23

ANSWER CASE 30

Answer: a

The differential of a left upper quadrant mass includes splenomegaly, and when it's large enough, it can reduce the stomach's ability to distend. When this occurs, the patient notices that small amounts of food result in a sensation of feeling full (early satiety). An enlarged spleen combined with a grossly elevated white cell count is suspicious of leukaemia. The white cell differential shows that the majority of the cells are mature myeloid. As the cells are maturing and the spleen has had time to enlarge to this extent, this is in keeping with chronic myeloid leukaemia (CML).

CML is associated with the Philadelphia chromosome t(9;22). A piece of chromosome 9 is translocated onto chromosome 22. The *BCR-ABL* gene is formed on chromosome 22. This results in a tyrosine kinase signalling protein always being turned on, resulting in uncontrolled cellular division.

This gene is used to diagnose the condition and also allows response to therapy to be assessed.

The treatment is with oral tyrosine kinase inhibitors including imatinib, dasatinib, nilotinib.

Note that the chromosomal abnormalities associated with haematological malignancies are acquired, rather than inherited and or congenital. This knowledge has facilitated an understanding of the oncogenesis underlying the development of the tumour cells and has also enabled more targeted therapies against the malignant cells, without damage to the bystander normal counterparts which don't have the abnormality.

Case 31

An 86-year-old attends primary care for a routine check-up. He is feeling well. His bloods have had a persistent abnormality for the past 10 years.

Hb 134g/L   (130–175)
WCC 16 × 10⁹/L   (4–11)
Neutrophils 3 × 10⁹/L
Lymphocytes 10 × 10⁹/L
Platelets 165 × 10⁹/L   (150–400)

To investigate the lymphocytosis, he underwent a CT chest, abdomen and pelvis that was unremarkable and had bloods sent for PB markers/immunophenotyping.

A B-cell clone was detected that was positive for CD5, CD23 and CD200 and negative for FMC7 and CD79.

Given the likely diagnosis, what would be an indication for treatment?

a) Weight loss 5% in 6 months
b) Weight gain
c) Lymphocyte doubling time of less than 6 months
d) Lymphocyte doubling time of 1 year
e) Recurrent chest infections

ANSWER CASE 31

Answer: c

The diagnosis is chronic lymphocytic leukaemia (CLL), which is a type of blood cancer. It generally progresses slowly, affecting the blood and bone marrow. It is more common in the elderly and characterised by an increase in lymphocytes.

The diagnosis can be made by a peripheral blood sample for flow cytometry. A B-cell clone $>5 \times 10^9$/L with a phenotype of CD5+, CD23+, FMC7–, CD79b– and weak light-chain restriction is typical. About 92% of patients with CLL present with a score 4 of 5 or 5 of 5.

Note that if the CLL score is lower and is CD5+, then the main differential is mantle cell lymphoma, and it usually is CD200– and characterised by t(11;14) chromosomal abnormality.

The majority of patients with CLL will not require treatment and although not curable, it can be so indolent that patients can live a normal life span.

It can cause problems requiring treatment:

If there is a large volume of disease in the bone marrow, then the normal bone marrow function can become impaired, for example, a progressive anaemia or thrombocytopenia.

If the lymphocyte doubling time is less than 6 months, this means that it has a more aggressive form and treatment is justified, as symptoms will arise.

Infections are not unusual in CLL, and the most common cause of death is infection. Patients are advised to monitor for signs/symptoms of infection and get antibiotics urgently. They should also be encouraged to keep all vaccinations up to date, including COVID, flu, RSV, pneumococcal and non-live recombinant shingles.

Case 32

A 62-year-old presented with a confirmed DVT in the right femoral vein. Bloods showed a persistently elevated platelet count with normal inflammatory markers and normal iron stores.

The JAK2V617F mutation has come back negative.

Which of the following is most likely?

a) MPL
b) JAK2 exon 12
c) CALR
d) TET2
e) No myeloid mutation detected

Answer: a

Thrombocytosis is an increase in the platelet count. This rise can be caused by iron deficiency and inflammatory causes. If the patient is iron replete with normal inflammatory markers and the thrombocytosis is persistent, then there should be concern for an underlying myeloproliferative disorder like essential thrombocytosis (ET).

This cancer is diagnosed by:

- Sustained platelet count >450 × 10⁹/L
- Bone marrow biopsy demonstrating proliferating megakaryocytes
- Not meeting criteria for another myeloproliferative disorder like CML, PV, PMF or MDS
- Presence of JAK2, CALR or MPL mutation

Mutations can now be found in 90% of cases (JAK2V617F 50%, CALR 30%, MPL 10%).

Case 33

A 75-year-old has had a 3-month history of generalised headaches, blurred vision and noticed an itch after the shower.

There is no past medical history of any heart or lung diseases and no smoking history.

On examination, the neurological examination is unremarkable.

Hb 204g/L   (130–175)
Hct 0.65
WCC 12 × 10⁹/L   (4–11)
Platelets 398 × 109/L (150–400)

What investigation is most likely to confirm the diagnosis?

a) JAK2V617F
b) JAK exon 12
c) CALR
d) MPL
e) BCL-ABL

DOI: 10.1201/9781003501190-37

ANSWER CASE 33

Answer: a

Patients with persistently raised haemoglobin/haematocrit should be investigated. As discussed in case 6, there are no obvious causes of a secondary polycythaemia like lung disease, history of obstructive sleep apnoea or smoking. This aquagenic itch should also raise concerns of primary aetiology. Over 95% of cases are JAK2V617F-mutation positive with a small number of JAK exon 12. There is no association with CALR, MPL or BCR-ABL mutations.

Case 34

A 65-year-old has undergone extensive investigations for weight loss and pancytopenia. CT chest, abdomen and pelvis has shown a spleen size of 25cm with no lymphadenopathy or metastatic cancers.

Hb 95g/L	(130–175)
WCC 6.5 × 10⁹/L	(4–11)
Platelets 75 × 10⁹/L	(150–400)

Blood film: Tear drop red cells seen, leucoerythroblastic

Bone marrow aspirate was a dry tap, and trephine section is awaited.

What is the most likely diagnosis?

a) Chronic myeloid leukaemia
b) Hodgkin lymphoma
c) Primary myelofibrosis
d) Metastatic renal carcinoma
e) Sepsis

ANSWER CASE 34

Answer: c

Myelofibrosis is a rare blood cancer characterised by scar tissue/fibrosis building up in the bone marrow. If it occurs in isolation, it is referred to as primary myelofibrosis (PMF). A complication of polycythaemia vera (PV) or essential thrombocytosis (ET) is that it can transform into myelofibrosis. This is known as secondary myelofibrosis. The mutations found in PMF have the same frequency as that of ET: JAK2V617F mutation 50%, CALR 30% and MPL 10%.

Prognosis with myelofibrosis is poor, and if the patient is symptomatic with splenomegaly, then JAK inhibitors like ruxolitinib can be started.

Case 35

A 65-year-old man presents with back pain; MRI spine demonstrated diffuse lyric bone lesions.

Hb 98g/L   (130–175)
CCa 3.7mmol/L   (2.2–2.6)
GFR 28mL/min/1.73m²   (>60)
Paraprotein 40g/L IgGK

What is the pathophysiological trigger involved in the development of the bone lesions?

a) Calcium is absorbed by myeloid blasts in the bone marrow
b) Prostate cancer directly invades and erodes the cortical bone
c) Plasma cells in myeloma activate osteoclasts via RANKL
d) Plasma cells in myeloma activate osteoblasts via IL-1b and bFGF
e) The urinary losses of calcium are extremely high, resulting in bone reabsorption to stabilise ionic calcium
f) Tumour results in localised dehydration of the marrow, creating pseudo lytic lesions on MRI

ANSWER CASE 35

Answer: c

Myeloma is a cancer of plasma cells and commonly associated with a paraprotein. Normal healthy plasma cells do not have the ability to divide. Their role is to make immunoglobin against a pathogen that the body has previously encountered (memory/adaptive response). Each plasma cell secretes a different immunoglobulin, and therefore, during inflammation or infection, a polyclonal rise in immunoglobulins is not unusual.

A malignant plasma cell secrets an identical immunoglobulin, and as the malignant plasma cells divide, they secrete even more identical immunoglobulin exponentially. This identical immunoglobulin is referred to as a paraprotein.

Myeloma is diagnosed when clonal plasma cells are >10% of nucleated bone marrow cells. If the % is >60% or if there is any related organ or tissue impairment (ROTI), this is classified as symptomatic myeloma and requires treatment.

ROTI includes (mnemonic CRAB):

- hyper**C**alcaemia
- **R**enal impairment
- **A**naemia
- lytic **B**one lesion (>1 focal lesion that's >5mm on MRI)

The pathophysiology of the bone lesions is through the RANK/RANKL/OPG system.

Smouldering myeloma is when there is >10% clonal plasma cells but <60% and no ROTI.

Monoclonal gammopathy of undetermined significance (MGUS) is more common as we age and is a premalignant disorder with 1% per annum risk of progression. IgM MGUS arises from B lymphocytes and therefore can arise/progress to lymphomas, and generally, the non-IgM (IgG, IgA, IgD, IgE) should be monitored for progression to myeloma.

MGUS is the presence of a paraprotein but <10% clonal plasma cells on bone marrow (serum paraprotein <30g/L) and no attributable organ damage.

Case 36

A 75-year-old man attended the ED after spontaneously fracturing his femur. An urgent CT chest, abdomen and pelvis was performed. It was noted the patient had widespread lytic lesions throughout his spine, pelvis and proximal ends of his long bones. His prostate looked enlarged, but there was no defined mass. The organs appeared unremarkable.

What is the likely diagnosis?

a) Metastatic prostate cancer
b) Plasma cell myeloma
c) Osteoporosis
d) Osteomalacia
e) Osteosarcomas

ANSWER CASE 36

Answer: b

Causes of sclerotic bone lesions:

- Osteosarcoma
- Metastases: Prostate, breast, kidney, thyroid, lung, testicles (think of the paired organs or the ones with 2 lobes)
- Infarcts
- Bone islands
- Osteopetrosis
- Paget's

Causes of lytic bone lesions:

- Myeloma
- Bone cysts
- Solid tumours can cause mixed sclerotic/lytic (but usually sclerotic)

If the bone imaging is suspicious of a sinister cause of bone lesions, then, after a thorough history, a CT C/A/P is useful to look for a primary cancer. Other investigations could include US testicles or breast mammography.

Lytic lesions should have a full myeloma screen, as 95% of cases secrete a paraprotein.

(FBP, U&E, paraprotein electrophoresis, serum free light chains [SFLC] and a bone profile)

Case 37

A 23-year-old presented to his general practitioner with tiredness and weight loss. On examination, he had a firm mass in the left supra clavicular fossa. Biopsy reported Reed–Sternberg cells with an infiltrate of small lymphocytes, eosinophils and polymorphs.

Given the likely diagnosis, what virus is associated?

a) EBV
b) CMV
c) *H. pylori*
d) HHV8
e) HIV

ANSWER CASE 37

Answer: a

Lymphoma is a type of cancer that primarily arises from the lymphatic system. The majority of cancers get more common as we age, and Hodgkin lymphoma does have a peak in older age, but interestingly, there is another peak in the late teenage years and early 20s.

There are over 70 different types of lymphoma. Patients can present in various ways, for example with lymph node swelling, coincidental findings on CT scans or with B symptoms. B symptoms include fever, drenching night sweats or unintentional weight loss of 10% in 6 months.

Lymphomas are classified by their microscopic appearance, supplemented by immunohistochemistry for sub-classification, and therefore, a good biopsy is essential. A lymph node excision is preferred over a core biopsy. A fine-needle aspiration is not useful to classify the lymphoma but can sometimes exclude a solid cancer that had spread to the lymphatic system.

Lymphomas are classified initially into Hodgkin and non-Hodgkin lymphoma. Classical Hodgkin lymphoma has a distinctive biopsy characterised by a large, sometimes binucleated cell surrounded by an inflammatory infiltrate of small lymphocytes, eosinophils and polymorphs. The Hodgkin cell is called a Hodgkin Reed–Sternberg cell (HRS). Epstein–Barr virus (EBV) is seen in 40% of Hodgkin biopsies.

A CT chest, abdomen and pelvis is useful to stage lymphomas but, if available, a CT PET can upstage a patient, as normal-sized lymph nodes may contain disease.

Lymphomas are staged by the Ann Arbor classification from I to IV depending on the amount of lymph nodes involved. Stage I is a single lymph node area. Stage II is 2 or more areas on 1 side of the diaphragm. Stage III is disease on both sides of the diaphragm, and stage IV is diffuse disease with the involvement of 1 or more extra-lymphatic organs or sites.

Hodgkin lymphoma is mainly treated with chemotherapy. For limited disease, the cycles of chemotherapy may be reduced and combined with radiotherapy.

If patients with Hodgkin lymphoma ever need blood transfusion, it must be irradiated.

Other microorganisms and cancer associations:

EBV	Burkitt's lymphoma, diffuse large B-cell lymphoma, Hodgkin lymphoma, gastric adenocarcinoma, nasopharyngeal cancer
Human papilloma virus	Types 16 and 18 cervical cancer, types 6 and 11 vulva cancer
Hepatitis B	Hepatocellular carcinoma
Hepatitis C	Hepatocellular carcinoma
Polyoma virus	Merkel cell skin cancer
Herpes virus	Kaposi's sarcoma, primary effusion lymphoma
Human T-lymphotrophic virus (HTLV)	Adult T-cell leukaemia
HIV	Lung, liver, anal, Kaposi, non-Hodgkin lymphoma, oropharyngeal cancer
H. pylori	Gastric cancer, mucosa-associated lymphoid tissue (MALT) lymphoma
S. haematobium	Bladder cancer

Case 38

A 45-year-old man attends with unexplained weight loss of 2 stone in 6 months. He has no significant past medical history. On examination, there is no appreciable organomegaly or abdominal masses. Lymph node examination has found a 3 cm mass in the left supraclavicular fossa. It is non-tender and has a smooth surface and a rubbery feel.

CT chest, abdomen and pelvis has also shown retro-peritoneal lymphadenopathy.

Ultrasound-guided core biopsy of the supraclavicular lymph node demonstrated diffuse sheets of centroblasts. The cells have a vesicular chromatin and membrane bound nucleoli.

What is the likely diagnosis?

a) Metastatic gastric cancer
b) Lung cancer
c) Hodgkin lymphoma
d) Non-Hodgkin diffuse large B-cell lymphoma
e) Infection

ANSWER CASE 38

Answer: d

Lymphadenopathy that is progressive and painless is concerning for an underlying malignancy. Cancers that arise from the lymphatic system are called lymphomas, and certain solid cancers can spread to the lymphatic system as they progress. Virchow's node is gastric cancer spreading to the lymph node in the left supra clavicular fossa. Scalene lymph node is located deep to the sternocleidomastoid muscle and can become involved with lung cancer. The examination for the lymph node can give a clue as to whether lymphoma or solid cancer is likely. Lymphocytes normally reside in the lymphatic system, and when they turn cancerous, the lymph node swells uniformly, giving a rubbery, smooth feeling. Solid cancers that spread to the lymph node grow in clumps similar to their native organ, causing the lymph node to have a craggy feel.

Irrespective of examination, a progressive lymph node needs to be imaged and, if suspicious, biopsied.

The biopsy is reviewed by a pathologist who examines the tissue with a standard H&E stain. The microscopic appearance usually gives a clue to the underlying diagnosis. This then allows further specific stains to be requested to confirm the diagnosis.

This case is lymphoma, as there are no Hodgkin cells seen, and the description is that of diffuse large B-cell lymphoma (DLBCL).

Non-Hodgkin lymphomas are divided into the cell type, B and T cell. Further sub-division occurs, and the B cells are divided into high-grade and low-grade lymphomas. In high-grade lymphomas like DLBCL, the cancer cells are awake and dividing quickly. If left untreated, prognosis can be a few months. However, as the cells are awake, they are sensitive to immunochemotherapy and respond well. Remission rates are in excess of 70%. On the other hand, low-grade lymphomas have dormant cells; the disease can stay dormant or progress. Unfortunately, given the dormant cells, they cannot be fully eradicated with immunochemotherapy and therefore not curable if beyond stage I.

Case 39

A 32-year-old man received his second cycle of chemotherapy for Hodgkin lymphoma 10 days ago. He felt unwell with high temperatures and had a recording at 39°C. He contacted the chemotherapy helpline and was advised to attend immediately for an assessment.

On arrival:

RR 25
Sats 92% BA
BP 100/70mmHg
HR 110BPM
T°C 39.5

Immediately oxygen was administered with IV fluids and paracetamol. Bloods were sent. Saturations are now 99%, HR 86BPM and temperature 37.1°C.

What is the next most important step?

a) Await results of bloods to determine best course of action
b) Transfer to ICU for close observation
c) Administer IV broad-spectrum antibiotics before blood results are available
d) Assess hourly urinary output, and if suspicion of infection on blood results, administer antibiotics accordingly
e) Suspect progressive lymphoma, organise CT chest, abdomen and pelvis

ANSWER CASE 39

Answer: c
It is important that both at-risk patients and healthcare practitioners recognise neutropenic sepsis. If unstable, then immediate transfer to the ED is crucial. If stable, then patients attend haematology or oncology outpatient for an immediate assessment.

Sepsis 6 bundle within the 1st hour:

1) Oxygen
2) Bloods, FBP, U&E, CRP, LFT, coagulation, blood gas including glucose and lactate, urinalysis, blood cultures, sputum O&S, CXR
3) Antibiotics: IV broad-spectrum—do not delay until neutropenia confirmed. Anti-pseudomonas cover is important with drugs like tazobactam (Tazocin)
4) IV fluids
5) Serial lactate measurements
6) Urinary output, fluid balance

Case 40

A 66-year-old patient attends with a progressive headache for 3 weeks. On examination, the face appears swollen, and there are collateral veins over the anterior chest wall. The patient has known COPD and smokes 40 packs a year.

What is the likely diagnosis?

a) SVC obstruction
b) Right-sided heart failure
c) Mycobacterium lung infection
d) Tuberculosis
e) Subarachnoid haemorrhage

DOI: 10.1201/9781003501190-44

ANSWER CASE 40

Answer: a

Superior vena cava obstruction (SVCO) is an emergency. This needs immediate discussion with the oncology team. The SVC can be compressed from a surrounding tumour like a bronchogenic carcinoma or a lymphoma.

If compressed, less blood is being returned to the heart, and therefore facial swelling, headache, arm swelling and distended veins can be seen over the anterior chest wall.

Imaging with a CT confirms the diagnosis, and a guided biopsy determines the cancer subtype.

Immediate treatment options include dexamethasone with PPI; depending on the type of cancer other options include chemotherapy, radiotherapy or stent insertion.

As the vein was compressed, there is an increased chance of thrombus formation, and if found, the patient may require anticoagulation.

Case 41

A 76-year-old presents with progressive tiredness over the past 9 months. There is no significant past medical history, no regular medications and no history of alcohol.

Hb 86g/L   (130–175)
MCV 106fL
WCC 3.2 × 10⁹/L   (4–11)
Platelets 105 × 10⁹/L   (150–400)
B12: Normal level
Folate: Normal
Thyroid function test (TFT): Normal

What would be the most likely diagnosis?

a) Hypothyroid
b) Haemolysis
c) Thalassaemia
d) Myelodysplasia
e) Iron deficiency

ANSWER CASE 41

Answer: d

This case is of a pancytopenia, but the most severely affected lineage is the degree of anaemia.

The anaemia is macrocytic, and therefore, causes include B12 deficiency, folate deficiency, hypothyroid, alcohol, drugs and myelodysplasia.

In this case the B12, folate, TFT are normal and there is no history of medications or alcohol.

This is therefore likely myelodysplasia. In MDS, the bone marrow does not make enough healthy blood cells. The diagnosis is made with a bone marrow biopsy, cytogenetics and molecular analysis. From these results, this cancer is classified into subtypes. It is important that this classification occurs, as different MDSs have different prognoses and risks of developing acute leukaemia. Some MDSs can be so mild they don't require any intervention; others may require blood product support and trials of EPO. High-risk MDS may even require chemotherapy similar to that for AML.

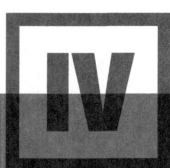

section IV

Laboratory Haematology Science

Case 42

A 75-year-old was admitted for an elective hip replacement.

Routine FBP:

Hb 123g/L   (130–175)
WCC 5.6 × 10⁹/L   (4–11)
Platelets 65 × 10⁹/L   (150–400)

Blood film: Platelet clumping
Coagulation screen: Normal

What is the next most appropriate step?

a) Proceed with hip replacement
b) Repeat EDTA platelet count
c) Delay operation until platelet count normal
d) Administer a platelet infusion
e) Start an anti-platelet drug

ANSWER CASE 42

Answer: a

To test an FBP, the blood is placed in blood bottle containing an anticoagulant, ethylenediaminetetraacetic acid (EDTA). The EDTA can activate platelets' surface glycoproteins, resulting in platelet activation and aggregation. Microscopic evaluation shows the platelets are clumped together. EDTA-dependent pseudo thrombocytopenia can occur, resulting in the analyser giving a falsely low platelet count.

The patient's platelet count is usually normal. The FBP can be repeated with another blood collection tube anticoagulant such as sodium citrate, which should show a higher platelet count.

In this case, the diagnosis is made from the blood film showing clumps. The platelet count is 65×10^9/L on the analyser but much higher in vivo. The procedure could proceed, as platelets are good enough. If the analyser was reading lower and more reassurance was required, a citrated platelet count could be performed.

When there is a true thrombocytopenia, most surgical interventions can occur with a platelet count $>50 \times 10^9$/L. However, when there is a CNS bleed or orbital, then a platelet count $>100 \times 10^9$/L is more appropriate, as these are high-risk areas in confined compartments.

Case 43

A 60-year-old lady presents with a cough, green sputum and dyspnoea over 1 week.

CXR demonstrates left upper lobe consolidation.

She has also complained of an intermittent headache.

Bloods:

Hb 78g/L   (130–175)
MCHC 370g/L   (320–360)
WCC 12.7 × 10⁹/L   (4–11)
PLT 345 × 10⁹/L   (150–400)
CRP 87mg/L   (<5)
Procalcitonin 3ng/mL   (<0.15)
Blood film: Red cell agglutination
DAT/Coombs   c3d positive

What is the unifying diagnosis?

a) Mycoplasma infection resulting in anti-I antibody
b) Streptococcal pneumonia with HSV activation
c) Infectious mononucleosis with anti-I antibody
d) Lower respiratory tract infection in a myeloma patient
e) Tuberculosis

ANSWER CASE 43

Answer: a

From the presentation, the patient has signs and symptoms of an infection. The high CRP and procalcitonin fit with the diagnosis. However, from the other bloods, we can see haemolysis.

The low Hb, high reticulocyte, high LDH and absent haptoglobins confirm haemolysis. The DAT/Coombs and blood film then give clues to the underlying aetiology. The red cell agglutination/clumping with the c3d positivity on the DAT suggests a cold agglutinin disease CAD.

CAD is caused by an IgM. The large pentameric IgM is able to cross over the negative charges on the red cells, resulting in the clumping of red cells together.

CAD IgM antibodies can be caused by infections like EBV, CMV, hepatitis and mycoplasma and lymphomas like Waldenstrom's, lymphoplasmacytic lymphoma and other B-NHL.

Certain cold antibodies can target specific antigens on the red cell surface. Mycoplasma infection can generate an anti-I, resulting in haemolysis and EBV with anti-I antibody.

Case 44

A 45-year-old man presented with necrotic fingers and toes. He has no significant past medical history, and bloods here done to investigate.

Hb 145g/L (130–175)
Platelets 1200 × 10⁹/L (150–400)—impedance method
Platelets 320 × 10⁹/L (150–400)—optical method
WCC 4.5 × 10⁹/L (4–11)
Vasculitis screen: Negative
Autoimmune screen: Negative
Blood film: Normal platelet numbers and morphological appearance; background stain shows precipitates of pale amorphous particles
No paraprotein detected.
CT chest, abdomen and pelvis: No lymphadenopathy or other malignancy seen

What is the most common trigger?

a) Hepatitis A
b) Hepatitis C
c) Myeloma
d) Leukaemia
e) Raynaud's

ANSWER CASE 44

Answer: b

The history suggests an issue with blood circulating to the peripheries. The clue to the aetiology in this case is the discrepancy in the platelet count with 2 different methods. This shows something in the plasma the same size as a platelet interfering with the impedance analyser and therefore tricking the machine into thinking they are platelets.

The blood film shows this material. However, to confirm the diagnosis, a cryoglobulin method should be performed.

Cryoglobulins are classified into 3 groups. Type 1 is a monoclonal immunoglobulin and can be associated with B-cell lymphomas. Type II and Type III are mixed cryoglobulins and can be associated with hepatitis C.

Case 45

A 22-year-old woman presented to the ED with acute-onset light-headedness and nausea. She recently started a course of dapsone.

On examination, cyanosis was noted, and the oxygen saturations were recorded at 85% despite the use of a non-rebreathing face mask.

CXR demonstrated no relevant findings.

An ABG was performed; blood was noted to be a chocolate brown colour and the methaemoglobin level was found to be 15%.

Within minutes of administration of methylene blue, the patient's cyanosis had resolved.

Which effect on the oxygen dissociation curve is correct?

a) Increase in 2,3 DPG moved the curve to the left
b) Decrease in pH moved the curve to the left
c) Methaemoglobin moved the curve to the left
d) Methylene blue moved the curve to the left
e) Decrease in CO_2 moved the curve to the right

ANSWER CASE 45

Answer: c

The oxygen dissociation curve is a useful way to understand how the blood carries and releases oxygen.

At high partial pressures of oxygen, haemoglobin binds to oxygen to form oxyhaemoglobin. At low partial pressures of oxygen in the tissues, the oxyhaemoglobin releases the oxygen.

The sigmoid shape arises because of cooperative binding. This is when haemoglobin with some oxygen already bound to its polypeptides has more of an attraction to get all 4 globin chains bound to oxygen (see Figure 45.1).

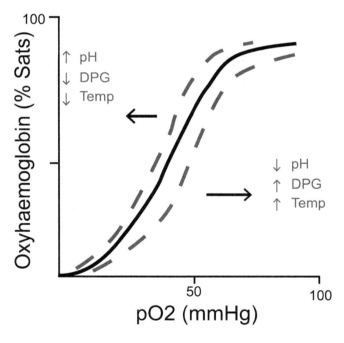

FIGURE 45.1 Oxygen dissociation curve shifts with changes in environment.

The mnemonic for remembering the factors that shift the curve to the right is CADET (think CADET RIGHT!), p**C**O$_2$; **A**cid; 2,3 **D**PG; **E**xercise; and **T**emperature. An increase in any of those factors moves the curve to the right.

Methaemoglobin is an abnormal form of haemoglobin in which the bound iron is no longer in its ferrous form but in ferric state. This results in a left shift in the oxygen dissociation curve as oxygen is held tight.

Case 46

A 42-year-old woman with rheumatoid arthritis is on methotrexate weekly. Unfortunately, due to a period of confusion, she was administered methotrexate daily. A progressive pancytopenia developed over the past 2 months.

Iron, B12 and folate levels are normal. Reticulocytes are 2%. As this is inappropriately low for the degree of anaemia, the patient was discussed with haematology.

What is methotrexate mode of action that results in pancytopenia?

a) Reduces folic acid absorption directly from the bowel
b) Inhibits dihydrofolate reductase, reducing levels of tetrahydrofolate
c) Changes cytosine nucleotide base to 5 methyl form, reducing its ability to pair with guanine
d) Increases tetrahydrofolate levels, blocking the availability of active folate
e) Potentiates the effect of dihydrofolate reductase, breaking down the availability of active folate

ANSWER CASE 46

Answer: b

Proliferating cells require the synthesis of DNA/RNA. Folate is an important analogue for DNA/RNA synthesis. Methotrexate (MTX) inhibits the enzyme dihydrofolate reductase, therefore depleting reduced folates and their availability for nucleotide base synthesis (see Figure 46.1).

MTX at high doses is used as a chemotherapy agent, in particular for CNS lymphoma.

High-cellular-turnover tissues like the skin, bone marrow and liver are sensitive to MTX; therefore, side effects include mouth ulcers, gastrointestinal intolerance, cytopenia and hepatitis.

If side effects need to be treated or drug levels are too high, then the fully reduced form of folate called folinic acid can be administered. This is independent of dihydrofolate reductase.

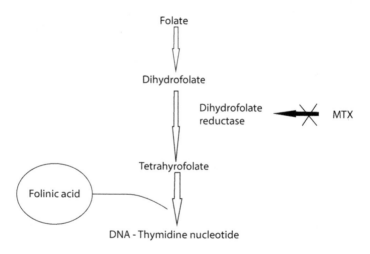

FIGURE 46.1 Folate metabolic pathway, demonstrating the effect of methotrexate inhibition of the enzyme dihydrofolate reductase.

Case 47

A 16-year-old man attended with jaundice and tiredness over the past few weeks. On further questioning, his mother informs you he had prolonged jaundice at birth but no other health concerns.

Hb 84g/L (130–175)
WCC 8.8 × 10⁹/L (4–11)
Platelets 258 × 10⁹/L (150–400)
LDH 532IU/L (70–250)
Reticulocytes 8% (1–2%)
Blood film: Spherocytes, polychromasia, bite cells
Haptoglobin: Absent
DAT/Coombs: Negative

What is the likely diagnosis?

a) Hereditary spherocytosis
b) Acquired warm autoimmune haemolytic anaemia
c) Zieve's
d) Glucose-6-phosphate dehydrogenase (G6PD) deficiency
e) Pyruvate kinase (PK) deficiency

ANSWER CASE 47

Answer: d

Glucose 6 phosphate dehydrogenase (G6PD) is an enzyme that protects your red blood cells from harmful oxidative stress. G6PD in the pentose phosphate pathway (PPP), which is quantitatively a small (9%) side branch of the metabolism of glucose to pyruvate/energy production for erythrocyte function. Glutathione (GSH) neutralises oxides and peroxides, forming a 2-glutathione-molecule form (glutathione disulphide, GSSG). The regeneration of reduced glutathione is brought about by the enzyme glutathione reductase, which converts NADPH to NADP+. G6PD is required to maintain a supply of NADPH and therefore glutathione to saturate oxygen free radicals (see Figure 47.1).

Normally, red cells can replenish the G6PD, but in patients with the genetic deficiency, unfortunately, exposure to triggers that increase oxygen free radicals can result in haemolysis. In these red cells, the

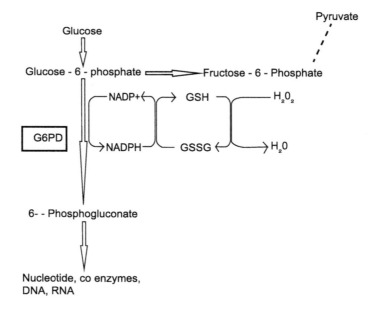

FIGURE 47.1 The important role of G6PD to maintain a supply of NADPH and therefore glutathione to saturate oxygen free radicals.

free radicals damage the haemoglobin, resulting in it clumping together (Heinz body). Once circulating through the spleen, there are attempts to remove the Heinz bodies by macrophages. Red cells can immediately lyse, resulting in anaemia and a positive haemolytic screen. Some red cells survive and circulate as bite cells.

Triggers include:

- Foods like fava beans
- Infections like CMV and hepatitis
- Many medications, including aspirin (high doses), vitamin K, nitrofurantoin, antimalarials, quinine and ascorbic acid. As so many medications are known triggers, once a susceptible patient is identified, it is important both the patient and the doctor try to avoid the triggers and, if not possible, to monitor for haemolysis.

G6PD deficiency is inherited as an X-linked recessive condition. Therefore, males are more likely to have G6PD deficiency because they only have 1 X chromosome. Some females may be affected if 1 or both copies of the G6PD gene are mutated. Females with 1 mutated gene may have lower G6PD activity and less risk of developing symptoms.

Enzyme testing to confirm diagnosis needs to wait until the acute haemolytic episode has resolved. During a crisis, the compensatory reticulocytosis can result in false normal G6PD levels, as reticulocytes carry more enzyme.

part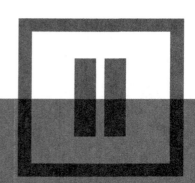

Additional Test Yourself Questions and Answers

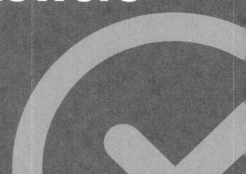

Test Yourself

1) **A 55-year-old man with a metal aortic valve attends for an INR check.**
   There are no signs of bleeding. His pulse rate is 70BPM, regular with a mechanical second heart sound.
   His INR is 5.1.

   What is the next step in his management?
   a) Administer 5mg vitamin K orally
   b) Hold a couple of doses of warfarin and monitor INR
   c) Continue the same dose of warfarin
   d) Administer prothrombin complex concentrate
   e) Administer 1–2mg warfarin

2) **A family has relocated to your area and now registered in primary care. The parents produce a medical letter informing you that all the children are homozygous HbSS. The family is aware that this condition can result in long-term morbidly and early mortality.**

   What is the most common cause of death in an affected adult?
   a) Sepsis
   b) Renal failure
   c) Stroke
   d) Cancer
   e) Haemosiderotic heart failure

3) **A 16-year-old attends the ED with priapism; it has been present for 8 hours, and symptoms of ischaemia are present. His FBP is normal, he has no paraprotein, denies any prescribed or illicit drugs. There is no history of trauma.**

What is the most likely cause?
a) Chronic myeloid leukaemia
b) Myeloma
c) Sickle cell anaemia
d) Aspirin
e) Thalassaemia

4) **A 39-year-old and her husband are from Taiwan. Both live an active lifestyle and are expecting their 1st child. Unfortunately, they missed their booking visit and presented to the antenatal team at 36 weeks in labour. Both parents' molecular diagnostic tests revealed 2 missing alpha genes in the cis chromosome.**
The child was born dead.

Given the likely diagnosis, what was pathophysiology attributing to the death?
a) $\gamma 4$ (gamma) bound O_2 tightly, resulting in poor tissue oxygenation
b) Sickling of red cells in cerebral vasculature
c) High levels of HbA2, retaining high levels of carbon dioxide
d) Reduced levels of beta chain, resulting in severe microcytic anaemia
e) Sepsis

5) **A pregnant 26-year-old in her 3rd trimester attends with a long history of tiredness. The patient has a history of iron deficiency and despite oral supplements continues to have a haemoglobin level of 100g/L. She is anxious this anaemia may be causing harm to the child.**

What is the best explanation that makes this unlikely?
a) The fetal blood volume is a lot smaller; therefore, iron deficiency has less of an effect
b) The predominant haemoglobin is fetal haemoglobin HbF; given the higher affinity, it can extract O_2 easily from maternal circulation
c) HbF has a lower affinity for oxygen, giving up oxygen readily to fetal tissue
d) HbF is made in fetal bone marrow, which has a large reservoir of stored iron
e) The fetus can tolerate severe anaemia without any harm

6) **A 65-year-old man presents with easy bruising, minor nosebleeds. It has only started in the last 2 years. His FBC and coagulation screen are within normal ranges.**

What cause is the most likely?
a) vWF disease
b) Congenital haemophilia
c) Acquired haemophilia
d) Prescribed anti-platelet medication
e) Ehler–Danlos syndrome

7) A 25-year-old from Indonesia attended for baseline bloods.

Hb 120g/L   (130–175)
MCV 63fL   (80–96)
Ferritin 80ng/mL   (30–400)
Iron saturation of 30%

What is the likely explanation of these blood results?
a)   Iron deficiency
b)   Sickle cell anaemia
c)   Alpha thalassaemia trait
d)   Beta thalassaemia major
e)   Hydrops fetalis

8) A 16-year-old attends with progressive tiredness.

Blood tests:
Hb 85g/L   (130–175)
MCV 111   (80–96)
WCC 4.5 × 10^9/L   (4–11)
Platelets 276 × 10^9/L   (150–400)

Which of the following may be the cause of these blood findings?
a)   Iron deficiency
b)   Folate deficiency
c)   Lead poisoning
d)   Thalassaemia
e)   Vit B6 deficiency

9) **A 16-year-old is awaiting spinal surgery. He is predicted to lose 6 units of blood. Pre-operative crossmatch has been performed. The lab contacts you to state that there will be a delay, as the patient is flagged for irradiated blood products.**

Which one of the following could be a reason why the products must be irradiated?
a) Age of patient
b) Previous transfusion reaction
c) History of Hodgkin lymphoma
d) Large volume of blood to be replaced
e) Previous exposure to radiotherapy

10) **A 23-year-old woman presents with widespread bruising.**

Blood tests:
Hb 123g/L   (130–175)
WCC 34 × 10⁹/L   (4–11)
Promyelocytes 15 × 10⁹/L
Blasts 10 × 10⁹/L
Platelets 50 × 10⁹/L   (150–400)
PT 28secs   (11.7–17.3)
APTT 56secs   (27–32)
FIB 0.8g/L   (1.5–4.5)

What genetic mutation is the likely cause?
a) t(15;17)
b) t(9;22)
c) t(11;14)
d) t(14;18)
e) t(8;14)

11) **A 75-year-old man was found on MRI to have numerous lytic lesions on his spine. His Hb was 101 g/L and GFR had dropped to 12 mL/min. His wife has noticed an increase in confusion, and the patient has been complaining of abdominal pain and constipation.**

What is the likely cause of the confusion?
a) Hypercalcaemia
b) Increased uric acid
c) Anaemia
d) Meningitis
e) Skull lytic lesion

12) **A coagulation result has come back with an isolated prolonged PT, normal APTT and normal fibrinogen.**

What is the cause of a prolonged PT?
a) FVIII deficiency
b) Factor X deficiency
c) Factor II deficiency
d) Factor VII deficiency
e) Factor V deficiency

13) A 32-year-old was found to have a platelet count persistently greater than 450 × 10⁹/L. There was no sign of infection, with a normal CRP, and iron stores are replete. Testing for essential thrombocytosis has shown no evidence of JAK2V617F mutation or CALR.

What is the next likely mutation?
a) JAK exon 12
b) BCR-ABL, t(9;22)
c) PML RARA, t (15;17)
d) TET2
e) MPL

14) A 85-year-old with a past medical history of hypertension and ischaemic heart disease suffered acute dyspnoea 2 hours after a blood transfusion. His JVP was elevated and bilateral creps heard on auscultation.

What is the most likely diagnosis?
a) TRALI
b) Acute haemolytic transfusion reaction
c) Pulmonary embolism
d) TACO
e) LRTI

15) A 51-year-old attended with progressive fatigue.

Blood tests:

Hb 75g/L	(130–175)
WCC 5.5 × 10^9/L	(4–11)
Platelets 234 × 10^9/L	(150–400)
Bilirubin 98μmol/L	(<21)
Indirect bilirubin 75μmol/L	
LDH 763IU/L	(70–250)
Haptoglobin: Not detected	
Reticulocytes 6%	(1–2)
DAT: IgG positive	

Which is the most appropriate treatment?
a) Transfusion support only
b) Rituximab
c) Prednisolone
d) Mycophenolate
e) Anti-D

16) A 65-year-old is diagnosed with a warm autoimmune haemolytic anaemia.

What are the expected blood film findings?
a) Red cell agglutination, polychromasia
b) Spherocytes, polychromasia
c) Schistocytes, thrombocytopenia
d) Tear drops
e) Bite cells

17) **A 75-year-old presented with a mass in the left supra clavicular fossa. It is painless and craggy on palpation. It does not transilluminate with light.**

What is the most likely diagnosis?
a) Cyst
b) Lymphoma
c) Infection
d) Tuberculosis
e) Gastric cancer

18) **A 65-year-old has had a 3-month history of generalised headaches, blurred vision and noticed an itch after a shower. There is no past medical history of any heart or lung diseases and no smoking history. His Epworth sleep score is low.**

On examination, the neurological examination is unremarkable.
Hb 204g/L   (130–175)
Hct 0.65   (0.42–0.45)
WCC 12 × 10⁹/L   (4–11)
Platelets 398 × 10⁹/L   (150–400)
The JAK2V617F mutation has come back negative.

What is the next likely mutation to cause this?
a) BCR-ABL
b) JAK exon 12
c) CALR
d) MPL
e) PML RARA

19) **A 65-year-old with non-valvular AF in currently on dabigatran. His last dose of medication was 5 hours ago. He was admitted with a 1-hour history of tiredness and profuse GI bleeding.**

On examination:
HR 150BPM
BP 75/30
Sats 94% BA
RR 22

What is the most suitable reversal agent?
a) FFP
b) Octaplex PCC
c) Idarucizumab
d) Andexanet alpha
e) Vitamin K

20) **A 22-year-old man had an emergency splenectomy 6 months ago.**

What would you expect to see on his blood film?
a) Blasts
b) Howell–Jolly bodies
c) Thrombocytopenia
d) Neutropenia
e) Bite cells

21) A 65-year-old attended with progressive fatigue and jaundice.

Blood tests:

Hb 65g/L	(130–175)
WCC 5.5 × 10⁹/L	(4–11)
Platelets 234 × 10⁹/L	(150–400)
Bilirubin 98μmol/L	(<21)
Indirect bilirubin 75μmol/L	
LDH 763IU/L	(70–250)
Haptoglobin: Not detected	
Reticulocytes 6%	(1–2)
DAT: c3d strongly positive	

What is the likely cause?
a) Warm autoimmune haemolytic anaemia
b) Cold autoimmune haemolytic anaemia
c) Liver disease
d) Gilbert's
e) Hereditary spherocytosis

22) A 29-year-old man is diagnosed with acute leukaemia.

What could you expect to see on his blood film to indicate the lineage is myeloid?
a) Blasts
b) Auer rods
c) Howell–Jolly bodies
d) Neutropenia
e) Bite cells

23) A coagulation result has come back with a prolonged PT, prolonged APTT and normal fibrinogen.

What could be a cause of this pattern?
a) FVIII deficiency
b) Factor IX deficiency
c) Factor XIII deficiency
d) Factor VII deficiency
e) Factor V deficiency

24) A 33-year-old man attended with progressive fatigue and jaundice.

Blood tests:
Hb 95g/L   (130–175)
WCC 5.5 × 10⁹/L   (4–11)
Platelets 234 × 10⁹/L   (150–400)
Bilirubin 98µmol/L   (<21)
Indirect bilirubin 75µmol/L
LDH 763IU/L   (70–250)
Haptoglobin: Not detected
Reticulocytes 9%   (1–2)
DAT: Negative
Blood film: Bite cells

Given the likely diagnosis, what could be a possible trigger?
a) Fava beans
b) Berries
c) Grapes
d) Walnuts
e) Apples

25) A 65-year-old man attended his GP for a check-up.

Hb 131g/L   (130–175)
CCa   2.5mmol/L   (2.2–2.6)
GFR >60mL/min/1.73m^2 (>60)
Paraprotein 2g/L IgGK
Skeletal survey: No lytic lesions

What is the likely cause of the paraprotein?
a)   Plasma cell myeloma
b)   Amyloid
c)   Waldenstrom's
d)   MGUS
e)   CLL

Test Yourself Answers

1 b
2 c
3 c
4 a
5 b
6 d
7 c
8 b
9 c
10 a
11 a
12 d
13 e
14 d
15 c
16 b
17 e
18 b
19 c
20 b
21 b
22 b
23 e
24 a
25 d

INDEX

Printed in the United States
by Baker & Taylor Publisher Services